D0417954

OXFORD HANDBOOKS IN EMERGENCY MEDICINE

1. The Management of Major Trauma
COLIN ROBERTSON AND ANTHONY D. REDMOND

The management of
Major Trauma

Colin Robertson
Consultant/Honorary Senior Lecturer in
Emergency Medicine, Royal Infirmary, Edinburgh

and

Anthony D. Redmond
Consultant in charge,
Accident and Emergency Service South Manchester

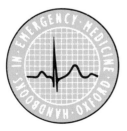

Oxford • New York • Tokyo
OXFORD UNIVERSITY PRESS
1991

Oxford University Press, Walton Street, Oxford OX2 6DP

Oxford   New York   Toronto
Delhi   Bombay   Calcutta   Madras   Karachi
Petaling Jaya   Singapore   Hong Kong   Tokyo
Nairobi   Dar es Salaam   Cape Town
Melbourne   Auckland

and associated companies in
Berlin   Ibadan

Oxford is a trade mark of Oxford University Press

Published in the United States
by Oxford University Press, New York

© Colin Robertson and Anthony D. Redmond 1991

British Library Cataloguing in Publication Data
Robertson, Colin 1953—
The management of major trauma.
1. Man. Trauma
I. Title   II. Redmond, Anthony D. (Anthony Damien)
617.21
   ISBN 0-19-261824-5

Library of Congress Cataloging-in-Publication Data
Robertson, Colin (Colin Ernest)
The management of major trauma/Colin Robertson and Anthony D. Redmond.
(Oxford handbooks in emergency medicine)
Includes index.
1. Wounds and injuries—Treatment.   2. Surgical emergencies.
3. Surgical intensive care.   I. Redmond, Anthony D.   II. Title.
III. Series.
[DNLM: 1. Emergencies.   2. Wound and Injuries—therapy.   WO 700 R649m]
RD93.R63   1991   617.1'026—dc20   90-7972 CIP
   ISBN 0-19-261824-5

Photoset by Cotswold Typesetting Ltd, Gloucester
Printed in Great Britain by
Biddles Ltd, Guildford and Kings Lynn

Preface

Trauma is the single commonest cause of death for individuals under the age of forty years, and the third commonest cause of death at all ages. These patients present to Emergency Departments with the most complex and challenging problems; and there is increasing evidence both in the United Kingdom and in North America that such cases are frequently mismanaged, with increased mortality and morbidity following as a consequence of delays, misdiagnosis, and mistreatment.

Yet such patients are often young and resilient, and if optimally treated should have a normal life expectancy. It is clear that the initial treatment such patients receive determines their ultimate outcome; and it is essential that this is rapidly and expertly provided.

It is a paradox in our system of health care in the United Kingdom, that the most seriously ill or injured patients are frequently dealt with by the most junior and inexperienced staff. There can be no substitute for experience, skill, adequate staffing-levels, facilities, and back-up.

Recognizing the current deficiencies in our system, this handbook is aimed at junior and middle-grade staff working in Accident and Emergency Departments faced with patients who have sustained multiple injuries. Middle-grade members of staff in related disciplines, such as general surgery, orthopaedics, neurosurgery, anaesthetics, and intensive care, who may be involved in the trauma team will also find areas directly applicable to their practice.

Of necessity, the resuscitation of such patients demands that a number of diagnostic and therapeutic techniques should be performed almost simultaneously on an individual patient. The text is arranged in sections relating both to initial resuscitation and to subsequent body-system examination and treatment. Each section is concluded by a list of 'key' points.

The style is deliberately didactic; but each section includes a list of suggested further reading. These references are not all-embracing, but will provide a depth of referencing and substantiation for the statements in the text. In addition, many of the references have themselves been chosen because they provide further extensive reference lists. This will enable those individuals wishing to undertake further studies, diplomas, or fellowships to access that information without difficulty. While the principles of major trauma management are identical for all ages, this book is primarily directed to adult patients. The specific problems associated with major trauma care in paediatric patients will be covered in a later volume in this series.

Edinburgh/Manchester   C.R.
1990   A.D.R.

Acknowledgements

Figs 1.1, 1.2, Tables 1.2 and 1.3 are adapted courtesy of the Office of Population Censuses and Surveys and HMSO.

Fig. 1.3. is reprinted by permission from the Transport and Road Research Laboratories Leaflet LF 762.

Table 1.1. is adapted from 'Injury in America' (1985) with permission from the National Academy Press, Washington DC and the Annual Report of the Registrar General for Scotland 1986.

Table 1.11. is reprinted from the Abbreviated Injury Scale 1985 Revision with permission of the Association for the Advancement of Automotive Medicine, Des Plaines, Illinois, USA.

Fig. 6.1. is reproduced from the ABC of Spinal Injury courtesy of British Medical Journal, and the Appendix figure is reproduced with permission from Flenley, D. C. (1971). *Lancet* **1**, 921.

In addition, we would like to thank Malcolm Gordon and David Steedman for their guidance and help in the production of **Fig. 4.1** and Professor J. D. Miller for the 'Indications for CT Scanning' in Chapter 3.

We are grateful to Daphne Lytton for the art work and illustrations of **Figs 10.1–10.19**.

Finally, we would like to thank Mrs Caroline Sinclair for help in the preparation of the manuscript, Dr Robin Illingworth for invaluable advice and support, and the Staff of the Oxford University Press for their encouragement and forebearance.

Contents

PART 1

General features of trauma and its primary management

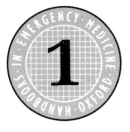

CHAPTER 1

The epidemiology and measurement of trauma

The epidemiology and measurement of trauma: a general introduction

• The scale of the problem   Financial cost   Prevention

In the developed world, trauma is the principal cause of death for both men and women under forty years of age, and it is the third commonest cause of death at all ages. In the United Kingdom, approximately 25 000 people are killed every year as a direct consequence of trauma, while a further 500 000 sustain major injury. The overall physical and emotional consequences of trauma are devastating for those injured, their families and friends, and the emergency services. Furthermore, at a time when the economics of health-care provision and efficiency are being carefully scrutinized, it is important to recognize the financial cost of trauma. It is currently estimated that the fiscal cost for one individual who dies as the result of a road-traffic accident in the United Kingdom is £500 000. In total, accidents consume approximately 1 per cent of a developed country's gross national product (approximately £3000 million annually in the United Kingdom).

It is not overstating the case to say that there is a trauma pandemic. Moreover, its impact is principally on the young members of society, and leads to a greater loss of working years of life than all forms of ischaemic heart-disease and neoplasia combined. In spite of this, the subject receives a tiny proportion of the total funding for research, in contrast to other conditions that kill mainly in later years.

Even within otherwise similarly developed countries there are marked differences in the rates of death from trauma and the mechanisms by which injury is sustained (Table 1.1). However, in all countries the biggest single contribution is made by road-traffic accidents. Road-accident rates are falling in the UK despite progressive rises in vehicular traffic; but nevertheless nearly 6000 deaths occur annually. Pedestrians, pedal cyclists, and motor-cyclists are particularly at risk; and the implementation and enforcement of safety measures is especially difficult for these groups (Tables 1.2 and 1.3).

Prevention is to be stressed as the only rational approach to

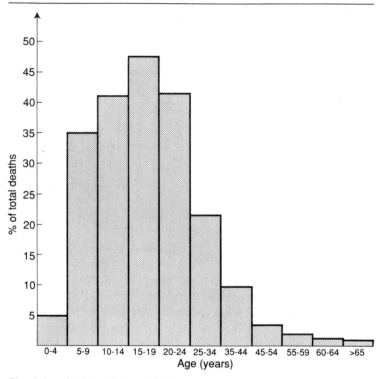

Fig. 1.1 • Accidental deaths from all causes as a proportion of total deaths by age-group

reduce the unacceptably high levels of mortality and morbidity. The three cornerstones of accident prevention are Education, Legislation, and Engineering. These three aspects should be interlinked, although particular emphasis may be required for specific situations. For example, young road-vehicle users appear to be relatively resistant to educational intervention, and so deterrent legislation and protective engineering are particularly important for this group.

Imaginative and enthusiastic education in schools can be highly effective, and must be encouraged; but it is much more difficult to change the attitudes of many adults in their perception of accident risk and prevention.

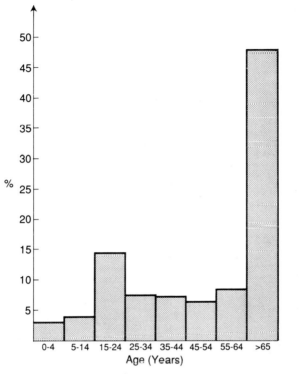

Fig. 1.2 ▪ Breakdown of all accidental deaths by age-group, UK 1985

Nationally, specific legislation covering the compulsory use of seat-belts, crash-helmets for motorcyclists, and drink-driving have had the most significant effects on road-traffic injury patterns; but considerably more is needed.

Following the introduction of compulsory seat-belt wearing by drivers and front-seat passengers of cars and light vans, deaths in these users fell by 18–25 per cent with similar reductions in the rates for serious injury. However, those groups at highest risk— the young, and those who have consumed alcohol—are least likely to comply with the requirement to wear seat-belts, and may therefore derive no benefit. Furthermore, many rear-seat passengers and children remain unprotected. It has been estimated

8 • The epidemiology and measurement of trauma

Table 1.1 • Deaths from injury: breakdown by causes, USA 1985 and Scotland 1986

	USA	Scotland
Road Traffic Accidents	30.3	30.1
Firearms	22.3	0.3
Falls	8.8	39.9
Drowning	4.9	3.3
Poisoning	4.9	1.1
Fires	4.0	7.5
Miscellaneous	24.8	17.8
	100.0%	100.0%

Table 1.2 • Casualties in road accidents (United Kingdom) 1985

Road user	Killed	Injured
Pedestrians	1848 (34.6%)	61 139 (19.1%)
Pedal cyclists	296 (5.5%)	27 077 (8.4%)
Motor cyclists and other two-wheeled motor-vehicle users	814 (15.2%)	56 459 (17.6%)
Car drivers	1307 (24.5%)	85 995 (26.8%)
Motor-vehicle passengers	935 (17.5%)	80 911 (25.2%)
Others	142 (2.7%)	9238 (2.9%)
Total	5342 (100%)	320 819 (100%)

Table 1.3 • Relative risk of death to road users in UK (rate per 100 million vehicle-kilometres)

Heavy-goods-vehicle drivers	1
Light-goods-vehicle drivers	1.5
Car drivers	2.5
Pedal cyclists	31
Motorcyclists	60

that up to 75 per cent of the 4000 UK deaths and serious injuries occurring annually in these categories could be prevented by wearing restraints. Without specific legislation no change in the perception of risk, and consequently of belt-use, on the part of these groups is likely.

The role of alcohol

• **Some statistics   Alcohol abuse   Associated effects   Educational programmes**

Up to 15 per cent of all patients attending an Emergency department, and about 10 per cent of all hospital in-patient admissions, occur as a direct consequence of alcohol abuse. Alcohol consumption per caput has risen steadily over the past forty years, and appears to be directly related to the cost of a unit of alcohol. Thus between 1945 and 1985 the annual consumption of alcohol per person rose by 21 per cent for beer, 306 per cent for alcoholic spirits, and 3082 per cent for wine. Alcohol misuse, with its attendant impact on trauma services, is widespread throughout the United Kingdom. Licensing laws appear to play only a very limited role in the control of alcohol consumption and misuse, though they can significantly affect the times of day at which the victims present following trauma.

There is no 'safe level' of blood-alcohol concentration in relation to its effects on impairment of concentration and function. Over twenty years have passed since the level of 80 mg of alcohol per dl of blood was chosen as the legal limit for drinking and driving in Britain. However, impairment of concentration and function can be detected at levels between 10 and 40 mg/dl. In addition, recent data suggest that drivers under the age of twenty or over the age of fifty-five have a particularly increased risk of accidents at these lower alcohol concentrations, and that the injuries then sustained are relatively more severe (Fig. 1.3). Acute alcohol intoxication increases morbidity and mortality in animals with haemorrhagic shock. In the few studies that have been performed in man, alcohol intoxication has been shown to double the mortality-rate for patients with acute head-injury. For road-traffic accidents,

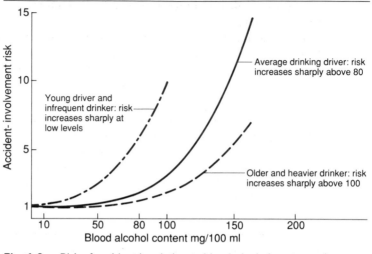

Fig. 1.3 • Risk of accident in relation to blood-alcohol concentration

33 per cent of all fatalities and 10 per cent of all injuries involve excess alcohol consumption; but it is not only those individuals involved in driving vehicles who contribute to these figures. Up to one-third of deaths among pedestrians are associated with alcohol, and of the 1500 UK road-deaths in which alcohol is directly implicated, approximately 480 intoxicated pedestrians, 625 intoxicated drivers, and 400 innocent victims die every year.

For other categories of trauma the role of alcohol is also depressingly great. Nearly one-fifth of people injured in the home have been drinking, as have up to 60 per cent of patients injured in assaults. For some other forms of traumatic death, alcohol appears to play an even greater role. Alcohol consumption is associated with over 50 per cent of the deaths from burns and fire-related injuries, 30 per cent of all drownings, 50 per cent of all homicides, and 25 per cent of fatal accidents in the workplace.

There is a direct link between violence and alcohol intoxication, and interestingly also between the severity of injury in victims of assault and the degree of their intoxication. Presumably recipro-cal aggression and loss of judgement induced by alcohol intoxication in the victim prolong the violent episode and also reduces the victim's capacity to avoid injury during the assault.

At present, alcohol abuse is probably the single most important cause of injury.

The implementation and impact of education programmes in this field have been hampered by gross under-funding in comparison with the vast sums spent upon advertising alcohol. Government inertia, together with the many vested interests involved in the use and sale of alcohol, serve only to cloud the complex issues further. Nevertheless, it is an important role for all concerned with trauma to address such problems, and to indicate where education, advice, and legislation should interact. If there is to be any improvement in the appalling toll that alcohol is currently taking, then major changes in public perception and attitudes will be required.

Pre-hospital management and transportation

• **Historical aspects   Trimodal distribution of deaths   Flying squads   On-scene care   Trauma Centres**

The concept of providing medical care at the scene of trauma was recognized by the ancient Greeks and Romans. In the first century special hospitals were established at sites of potential major conflicts to provide care for wounded legionaries. It was not, however, until the Napoleonic Wars that pre-hospital care took on recognizably modern forms.

Dominic Jean Larre, Napoleon's Surgeon-in-Chief, clearly understood the requirement for rapid evacuation and early surgical care for wounded soldiers, and was able to show dramatic improvements in the morbidity and mortality of patients thus treated. More recently, military experience has shown the benefits of providing immediate basic medical care with rapid evacuation to a facility able to provide definitive surgical care.

Overwhelmingly, the message from such experience has been that mortality is directly related to the time taken for a patient to reach such definitive surgical treatment. As, however, with many medical lessons learned in wartime, the application of these observations to civilian practice has been slow.

In the United States Trunkey and others have shown that death following civilian trauma has a trimodal distribution when mortality is plotted as a function of time following injury. The first peak comprises the 50 per cent of individuals who will die within thirty minutes of the event. For these patients death is due to such complex and severe injuries that survival is often impossible within the constraints of our current knowledge and technology. Typical examples would be those deaths resulting from major brain or brain-stem lacerations or massive vascular disruption within the thorax. In the absence of a 'medical' role, the principal concern for this group of patients must be to direct efforts towards accident-prevention.

The second peak, accounting for 30 per cent of all trauma deaths, occurs within four hours of injury. These deaths are characterized by major losses of circulating blood-volume, and are frequently compounded by a failure to provide and maintain an adequate airway and ventilation. The contribution of these components in producing death varies; but it has been estimated that up to 40 per cent of all patients in this group die as a consequence of airway obstruction, and up to 25 per cent have potentially correctable circulating-volume loss.

The third peak, 20 per cent of all trauma deaths, includes those patients who die days or weeks following trauma. This is commonly as a result of multiple organ failure, sepsis, or pulmonary embolism. Although such deaths usually occur in Intensive Therapy Units, there is evidence that with rapid, aggressive resuscitation and competent early surgical intervention mortality can be reduced within this third group.

It must not necessarily be assumed that experience of civilian or military trauma elsewhere in the world is directly relevant to the situation in the United Kingdom. Military experience involves young, fit individuals, whereas our trauma involves a spectrum of ages, with clusters in the third decade and among the over-60's. Similarly, in the USA up to 20 per cent of major trauma cases are related to penetrating injury from knife wounds and gunshots; but these problems are fortunately rare in the UK.

Knowing the contribution of volume-loss and airway problems to both early and late trauma deaths, it would appear from first principles that advanced airway care and volume-replacement in the pre-hospital phase would increase survival and reduce morbidity. Where there is delay, for example because of entrapment in road-vehicle accidents, this may be true. Prolonged entrapment for more than 10–15 minutes is, however, increasingly uncommon, despite the frequency of high-speed motor-vehicle collisions. With currently available cutting and release equipment appropriately co-ordinated rescue services should normally be able to release an entrapped victim from a vehicle in less than fifteen minutes. Operational constraints can also dictate the need for advanced pre-hospital trauma techniques: these may for instance be the result of delays in evacuating the injured to hospital because of geographical, environmental, or contamination difficulties. Our experience is that patients who cannot be rapidly evacuated to the receiving hospital must have special attention to airway patency, ventilation, volume-replacement, pain-relief, and splintage. This may be achieved by extended trained ambulance personnel, or by experienced medical 'Flying Squad' teams. Situations involving emergency amputation or major surgical intervention are now extraordinarily rare. This is partly as a consequence of improvement in the cutting and lifting equipment carried by the rescue services, but also because the above measures may permit stabilization of the patient even before full release and extrication.

In parts of the United Kingdom advanced pre-hospital trauma care is provided by hospital-based 'Flying Squads'. Studies have shown that in a small but significant proportion of such trauma cases mortality can be reduced by the intervention and activities of such flying squads. The use of AIS/ISS scoring and TRISS methodology (see p. 15) enables objective analyses of the value of flying squads.

These squads are, however, limited to large, usually teaching, hospitals that can provide experienced senior medical and nursing cover instantly twenty-four hours a day, seven days a week. Despite this, such squads are expensive neither to equip nor to run, and all centres which regularly provide such services agree that they are useful and necessary.

In other, often more remote, areas where advanced pre-hospital trauma care is required, schemes run by the British Association for Immediate Care (BASICS) provide a similar service. While ambulance crews trained and equipped to an advanced level are of clearly defined value in acute cardiac care, trauma is different. Within an urban or semi-urban environment, over 80 per cent of emergency patients can be transported to a major receiving hospital within thirty minutes of the initial call. Data from a number of sources have shown that to establish adequate intravenous access and give volume-replacement greater than 1000 ml exceeds site-to-hospital transit times, and thus leads to further delays in achieving appropriate in-hospital surgical resuscitation. For patients in Trunkey's 'early' death group who will die from blood-loss within four hours of injury, rates of blood-loss of 100–150 ml per minute are usual, and such losses cannot be adequately managed out of hospital. Similarly in the case of airway techniques the provision of advanced care is likely to be most valuable for those patients who have altered consciousness as a consequence of head-injury. But it should be recognized that those patients with head-injury accompanied by apnoea are extremely unlikely to have any favourable outcome; while, for the remainder, achieving endotracheal intubation will be at the cost of further temporal delays and the possibility of causing or exacerbating spinal injury. Furthermore, the opportunity for an individual ambulance crew-member to use such skills out of hospital will not be sufficiently frequent to maintain an adequate standard of competence.

The emphasis must therefore be on basic airway management, involving positioning and suction together with appropriate splintage and pressure techniques for external blood-loss. For those clinical situations involving delay where mass casualties are involved or where environmental or geographical locations pre-empt prompt evacuation, advanced pre-hospital trauma techniques may then be required, usually provided from the base-hospital. While the increasing use of helicopter transportation to reduce response-delays and facilitate evacuation from the scene is to be commended, it should not be thought of as the only aspect of this care that is required.

The most important point of all is that one must condemn the notion that trauma patients should be taken to the nearest hospital irrespective of the facilities available there. The North American and West German experiences are invaluable in this area. A series of meticulously performed and well-corroborated studies have shown that when major trauma cases are primarily directed to a designated regional Trauma Centre, preventable deaths can be cut by 80 per cent. The provision of the entire 'package' of trauma care, including pre-hospital, emergency department, and in-hospital phases, is central to such good results.

Recent studies in the UK confirm previous North American estimates that up to one-third of deaths following trauma are preventable. For patients with no injury to the central nervous system up to 60 per cent of deaths are avoidable. It is deeply worrying that in the UK up to 2500 injured patients per year reach hospital, but then die from potentially remediable conditions. The establishment of regional trauma centres in the United States has invariably led to a marked fall in preventable deaths. Concern that, as a consequence of this regionalization, longer transport times from the scene of the accident to the designated trauma centre may increase the death-rate has not been shown to be valid. Of greater import is the ability of the receiving hospital to provide, on an immediate basis, senior experienced staff who can provide multi-disciplinary care. Accident and Emergency Departments have a role in leading other disciplines to provide this standard. The provision of adequate diagnostic and therapeutic facilities is essential. The response-times for anaesthetic and surgical teams have been clearly demonstrated to be of crucial importance for the subsequent outcome.

Methods of assessing the severity of injury

• **Trauma Score   Revised Trauma Score   AIS and ISS scoring   TRISS methodology**

The ability to classify injuries and their sequelae objectively is central to the evaluation of the delivery of trauma care. This applies both to individuals and to groups of patients in whom the effects of preventive measures and treatments upon morbidity and mortality can be assessed.

Although attempts have been made from the very earliest times to classify injuries, these methods were often simplistic and non-reproducible, and failed to correlate closely with either individual or collective outcomes.

Two principal categories of assessment system have developed. The first of these consists of scales using readily available physiological measurements. The easiest and most widely applied physiological scoring system in international use is the Trauma Score (TS) first described by Champion in 1981. It uses the physiological parameters of systolic blood-pressure, capillary refill, respiratory rate and expansion, and the Glasgow Coma Scale. Specific ranges for each parameter are assigned coded

Table 1.4 · Scoring of the Trauma Score and the Glasgow Coma Scale

		Score
Trauma Score		
Respiration/min	≥36	2
	25–35	3
	10–24	4
	1–9	1
	None	0
Respiratory expansion	Normal	1
	Shallow	0
	Retractive	0
Systolic blood pressure, mm Hg	≥90	4
	70–89	3
	50–69	2
	0–49	1
	No pulse	0
Capillary return	Normal	2
	Delayed	1
	None	0

Table 1.4 • Scoring of the Trauma Score and the Glasgow Coma Scale

		Score	
Glasgow Coma Scale			
Eye opening	Spontaneous	4	Contribution of Total
	To voice	3	Glasgow Coma Scale Points to
	To pain	2	Trauma Score
	None	1	14–15=5
Verbal response	Oriented	5	11–13=4
	Confused	4	8–10=3
	Inappropriate words	3	5–7−2
	Incomprehensible words	2	3–4=1
	None	1	
Motor response	Obeys command	6	
	Localizes pain	5	
	Withdraw (pain)	4	
	Flexion (pain)	3	
	Extension (pain)	2	
	None	1	
Total Trauma Score		1–16	

values, and, when summated, the total Trauma Score can range between 1 and 16. As the physiological disturbances associated with the severity of injury increase, so the TS falls. This is demonstrated in Table 1.5, where the probability of survival (Ps) is given for each Trauma Score value between 1 and 16. By implication a fall in TS, for example in transit to hospital, indicates increasing physiological disturbance and greater risk of death.

Table 1.5 • Trauma score and probability of survival

Trauma Score	Probability of Survival (PS)
16	99%
15	98%
14	95%
13	91%
12	83%
11	71%
10	55%
9	37%
8	22%
7	12%
6	7%
5	4%
4	2%
3	1%
2	0%
1	0%

Interestingly, blood-pressure was not originally included as one of the TS parameters. This was because statistical analysis revealed that it was a poor predictor of outcome. However, early pilot studies showed that doctors would not complete a form which excluded blood-pressure, regardless of statistical consequences!

The Trauma Score has been used as a method of triaging patients in pre-hospital situations, and also of assessing the value or otherwise of specific interventions in the field prior to hospital reception. Further refinements of the system have produced the more recent Revised Trauma Score (RTS), which evolved from a critical analysis of patients studied in the recent North American Major Trauma Outcome Study (MTOS). In particular, by permit-

Table 1.6 • Revised Trauma Score

Glasgow Coma Scale	Systolic blood pressure (mm Hg)	Respiratory rate (min)	Coded value
13–15	>89	10–29	4
9–12	76–89	>29	3
6–8	50–75	6–9	2
4–5	1–49	1–5	1
3	0	0	0

Table 1.7 • Weights for Revised Trauma Score

Glasgow Coma Scale	0.9368
Systolic blood pressure	0.7326
Respiratory rate	0.2908

ting weighting of various aspects such as the Glasgow Coma Scale, severe head-injury can be identified in the absence of coexistent injury elsewhere. These revisions have resulted in more reliable predictions of patient outcome being achieved. However, if the RTS is used as a triage tool, its application is fundamentally different from that of the TS. Paramedics in the US who use the TS for triage purposes act in the recognition that a TS total of 13 or less indicates a mortality of greater than 10 per cent and accordingly evacuate such patients to a predesignated Level 1 Trauma Centre. If, however, the RTS is used for a similar purpose, instead of a numerical total being used to define this high-risk group, a trauma patient with a coded value of less than 4 in any of the three parameters is directed to the Level 1 Centre.

Although the TS and RTS are the most widely used and reliable of the currently available physiological scoring systems, they do have deficiencies. Up to 20 per cent of patients with severe injury may not be initially identified, usually because adequate physiological compensation has occurred or the assessment has been performed so rapidly following injury that detectable physiological compromise has not had time to occur. In addition, they may over-estimate the severity of injury when physiological changes

Table 1.8 • Sample patient (25-year-old male motorcyclist on arrival in A/E department)

		RTS coded values	RTS weighted
Resp. rate	30/min	3	2.1978
BP	85/30 mmHg	3	0.8724
G.C.S. E2.V2.M.5=	9/15	3	2.8104
RTS=			5.8806

occur which are not reflected in the measured parameters. Furthermore, these scores have not been validated for the very young or old.

The second group of techniques used for assessing the severity of injury are those based on the recognition and categorization of specific anatomical injuries in an individual patient. This information is available from the medical records, from data from operative findings, and at post-mortem.

In an attempt to establish a uniform rating system and to standardize the language used to describe injuries, the Abbreviated Injury Scale (AIS) was developed and published in 1971. Subsequent revisions have lead to the most recent version containing more than 1200 separate injury-descriptions, and this is the most widely used anatomical scale currently available for rating the severity of injury.

The Abbreviated Injury Scale describes specific injuries in an individual patient, which are each assigned a single code number on a scale of 1–6 (see Table 1.10). Injuries are grouped by body region and within each region injury-descriptions are listed in the AIS dictionary (see sample page from AIS dictionary, Table 1.11). The Abbreviated Injury Scale enables ranking of injury severity, but is non-linear with respect to the coded values and the severity of the injury sustained by the patient as a whole. It therefore has limitations when applied to patients with multiple injuries, as it is not possible to derive arithmetic mean values.

However, the AIS can be used to derive the Injury Severity Score (ISS). The ISS was initially based on an analysis of road-traffic accident victims in Baltimore by Baker and her colleagues, and for

Table 1.9 • Example of use of TS and RTS (25-year-old male motorcyclist involved in RTA; recordings taken on arrival in Emergency Department

Physiological parameters		Trauma Score	Revised Trauma Score (coded value)	RTS weights
Pulse:	128/min	—		
BP:	85/30 mmHg	3	3	$3 \times 0.7326 = 2.1978$
Respiratory rate:	30/min	3	3	$3 \times 0.2908 = 0.8724$
Respiratory expansion:	Retractive	0		
Capillary filling:	Delayed	1		
Glasgow Coma Scale:				
Eye opening:	To pain	2		
Verbal response:	Incomprehensible words	2		
Motor response:	Localizes pain	5		
	(Total GCS=9)	3	3	$3 \times 0.9368 = 2.8104$
		TS = 10		RTS = 5.8806

Table 1.10 · Abbreviated Injury Scale

AIS code:	Description
1	Minor
2	Moderate
3	Serious (non-life-threatening)
4	Severe (life-threatening—survival probable)
5	Critical (survival uncertain)
6	Unsurvivable (with current treatment)

the purpose of injury-severity scoring, the body is divided into six regions (see Table 1.12). An AIS code is assigned to each injury, and the ISS is calculated by summing the squares of the highest AIS codes in each of the three most severely injured body regions. Since the maximum score for any one region is 25, the highest possible ISS is 75 $((5 \times 5) + (5 \times 5) + (5 \times 5) = 75)$. Any patient with an injury severe enough to attract an AIS code of 6 in any one region is automatically awarded an ISS of 75.

The Injury Severity Score correlates closely with mortality, and is accepted world-wide as the 'gold standard' for the anatomical description of injury severity. Currently, major trauma is defined as a patient with an ISS score of 16 or more. This value predicts those patients with a greater than 10 per cent chance of mortality, and correlates with a Trauma Score of 13 or less. It also correlates well with length of hospital stay, but is much less accurate in predicting morbidity and in identifying long-term disability.

As with the physiological scoring systems, anatomical scoring has areas of deficiency. The initial versions were able to predict accurately the severity of injury and mortality in patients with blunt trauma, but were less accurate for penetrating injuries. The most recent update of the AIS dictionary (*AIS 90*) has incorporated penetrating injury, and has reduced this difficulty considerably.

The effect of age on the outcome of injury can also be incorporated into the assessment of the severity of injury. Generally speaking, for a given Trauma or Injury Severity Score, mortality increases with increasing age. In the United Kingdom, Bull, using probit analysis, has derived LD50 values for different age-groups based on the ISS.

Table 1.11 · Coded description of injuries to the neck

Injury description	Code
Whole area	
Decapitation	40101.6
Skin (includes all external skin and subcutaneous injury) [see EXTERNAL]	
Penetrating injury	
NFS	40102.2
no organ involvement	40103.2
complex with tissue loss/organ involvement	40104.3
Nerves	
Brachial plexus [see SPINE]	
Cervical spinal cord or nerve root [see SPINE]	
Vagus or phrenic injury	40201.2
Vessels	
Carotid (common, internal, external) artery	
NFS	40301.3
intimal tear no description	40302.3
with neurologic deficit not head related	40303.4
laceration	
NFS	40304.3
minor (superficial)^m	40305.3
with neurologic deficit not head related	40306.4
major^n (transection, rupture)	40307.4
with neurologic deficit not head related	40308.5
with segmental loss	40309.5
with thrombosis secondary to trauma	40310.3
with neurologic deficit not head related	40311.4

^{m} *Minor (superficial) = subtotal transection without major bleeding.*
^{n} *Major (rupture, transection) = major bleeding (approx. 1000 cc blood loss).*

Table 1.12 · Body regions used in ISS

1. Head and neck
2. Face
3. Chest
4. Abdominal/Pelvic Contents
5. Extremities/Pelvic Girdle
6. External, i.e. skin

Table 1.13 • Examples of AIS:ISS scoring techniques (25-year-old motorcyclist (see Tables 1.8 and 1.9)

Injury description	AIS code	ISS region
Concussional head injury (amnesia for accident, no neurological deficit)	2	Head/Neck
Fractures of 3rd to 9th ribs L chest with associated flail segment, and 700 ml haemothorax	_4_	Chest
Splenic rupture, 1200 ml haemoperitoneum at laparotomy	_3_	Abdomen/Pelvic contents
Minor laceration to small bowel mesentery	2	Abdomen/Pelvic contents
Closed fracture mid-shaft L femur	_3_	Extremities/Pelvic girdle
Compound displaced fracture mid shaft L tibia and fibula	3	Extremities/Pelvic girdle
Superficial abrasions to both hands and L elbow	1	External

$ISS = (4^2 + 3^2 + 3^2) = (16 + 9 + 9) = 34.$

The most refined and potentially useful application of both physiological and anatomical scoring is an integrated combination of Trauma and Injury Severity Scoring called the TRISS methodology (Trauma score, ISS, age combination index). This allows comparisons to be made between predicted and actual patient outcomes. Using the TRISS technique, the probability of survival (Ps) for any individual trauma patient can be calculated from the equation

$$Ps = \frac{1}{(1 + e^{-b})}$$

The constant $e = 2.718282$ (the base of Napierian logarithms), b is the sum of weighted coefficients derived from Walker–Duncan regression analysis carried out on over 30 000 severely injured patients in North America, and applied to the measured variables in this study. Age, above or below fifty-four years, and blunt or penetrating injury are weighted appropriately.

Table 1.14 · Revised TRISS methodology

$$Ps = \frac{1}{1+e^{-b}}$$

$$b = b_0 + b_1(RTS) + b_2(ISS) + b_3(A)$$

	b_0	b_1	b_2	b_3
Blunt	−1.2470	0.9544	−0.0768	−1.9052
Penetrating	−0.6029	1.1430	−0.1516	−2.6676

b coefficients are derived from analysis of MTOS data.

e = 2.718282 (the base of Napierian logarithms)

A is a variable related to patient's age:
if ⩽54 years A = 0; if >54 years A = 1.

TRISS techniques offer an objective approach to determining patient outcome, and also a uniform approach by which individual units can assess their own competence over periods of time and compare their results with those of other hospitals.

TRISS can be used graphically as a method of pin-pointing unexpected patient outcomes. Values of Trauma Score and ISS can be plotted in the form of a scatter diagram. A 50 per cent probability of survival (LD50) for a group of patients can be illustrated by a diagonal line as shown in Fig. 1.4. Survivors above

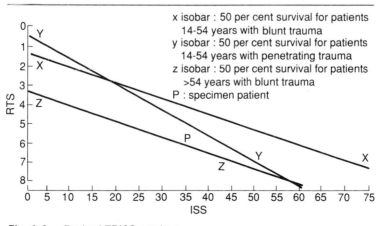

x isobar : 50 per cent survival for patients 14-54 years with blunt trauma
y isobar : 50 per cent survival for patients 14-54 years with penetrating trauma
z isobar : 50 per cent survival for patients >54 years with blunt trauma
P : specimen patient

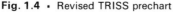

Fig. 1.4 · Revised TRISS prechart

the line and patients dying below the line are those with unexpected outcomes. Further investigation is then needed in the unit providing the trauma care to understand why these results have occurred and correct any deficiencies.

Table 1.15 • Calculation of probability of survival using revised TRISS technique

---

Example: 25-year-old motorcyclist, blunt injury
Revised Trauma Score 5.8806
Injury Severity Score 34

Probability of Survival (Ps) $= \dfrac{1}{1+e^{-b}}$

$b = b_0 + b_1(RTS) + b_2(ISS) + b_3(A)$

$b = [-1.2470] + [0.9544(5.8806)] + [-0.0768(34)] + [-1.9052(0)]$

$b = [-1.2470] + [5.6124] + [-2.6112] + [0]$

$b = 1.7542$

$Ps = \dfrac{1}{1+e^{-1.7542}}$

$Ps = \dfrac{1}{1+0.17304}$

$Ps = 0.8525$

Further reading

American Association for Automotive Medicine (1985). *Abbreviated Injury Scale: 1985 revision.* The Association, Arlington Heights, Illinois.

Anderson, I. D., Woodford, M., de Dombal, F. T., and Irving, M. (1988). Retrospective study of 1000 deaths from injury in England and Wales. *British Medical Journal,* **296**, 1305–8.

Anderson, I. W. R., Black, R. J., Ledingham, I. McA., Little, K., and Robertson, C. E. (1987). Early emergency care: the potential and benefits of advanced pre-hospital care. *British Medical Journal,* **294**, 228–31.

Baker, S. P., O'Neill, B., Hadden, W., and Long, W. B. (1974). The injury severity score. *Journal of Trauma*, **14**, 144–150.

Boyd, C. R., Tolson, M. A., and Copes, W. S. (1987). Evaluating trauma care: the Triss method. *Journal of Trauma*, **27**, 370–8.

Champion, H. R., Sacco, W. J., Carnazzo, A. J., Copes, W., and Forty, W. J. (1981). Trauma score. *Critical Care Medicine*, **9**, 672–6.

Dark, P., Little, K., Steedman, D., Gordon, M., and Robertson, C. (1990). An objective analysis of an Accident Flying Squad. *Scottish Medical Journal*, **35**, 73–6.

Foster, G. R., Dunbar, J. A., Whittet, D., and Fernando, G. C. A. (1988). Contribution of alcohol to deaths in road traffic accidents in Tayside 1982–1986. *British Medical Journal*, **296**, 1430–2.

Irving, M. (1981). Care of emergencies in the United Kingdom. *British Medical Journal*, **283**, 847–9.

Morris, J. A., Averbach, P. S., Marshall, G. A., et al. (1986). The trauma score as a triage tool in the prehospital setting. *Journal of the American Medical Association*, **256**, 1319–25.

Robertson, C. E. and Steedman, D. J. (1985). Are accident flying squads really cleared for "take-off"? *Lancet*, **ii**, 434–6.

Royal College of Surgeons of England. Working Party on the Management of Patients with Major Injuries (1988). *Report*. The College, London.

Shackford, S. R., Mackersie, R. C., Hoyt, D. D., et al. (1987). Impact of a trauma system on outcome of severely injured patients. *Archives of Surgery*, **122**, 523–7.

Spence, M. T., Redmond, A. D., and Edwards, J. D. (1988). Trauma audit— the use of Triss. *Health Trends*, **20**, 94–7.

Steedman, D. J. and Robertson, C. E. (1987). Who scores in trauma? *Care of the Critically Ill*, **3**, 77.

Trunkey, D. D. (1983). Trauma. *Scientific American*, **249**, 20–7.

Westaby, S. (ed.) (1988). *Trauma. Pathogenesis and treatment*. Heinemann, London.

Yates, D. W., Hadfield, J. M., and Peters, K. (1987). Alcohol consumption of patients attending two A/E departments in N.W. England. *Journal of the Royal Society of Medicine*, **80**, 486–9.

CHAPTER 2

Initial reception, clinical assessment, and resuscitation

Initial reception and clinical assessment: a general introduction

The initial reception, assessment, and emergency treatment of patients with multiple injuries must be a co-ordinated, simultaneous approach by an experienced team.

On arrival in the Emergency Department the patient should be admitted directly to the Resuscitation Area, while a doctor takes control of the airway, head, and neck. The initial phase of resuscitation will require two to three doctors and two experienced nurses per patient. This team must have a clearly identifiable, senior, experienced leader, and the team should work directly to his/her instructions.

The trolley on which the patient is placed must have tilt facilities and portable oxygen, and must permit radiographic examination of the patient without further movement.

All the patient's clothing must be removed (including underclothes), usually with scissors, to ensure adequate access to and examination of the patient.

The principles involved in the initial assessment of such patients are as follows:

- to identify and correct immediately life-threatening conditions;
- to ensure that second 'accidents' do not occur, by preventing any further deterioration in established conditions;
- to institute those treatments which can commence before definitive diagnosis; and
- to complete and act upon those investigations which will alter the immediate management of the patient.

The examination and treatment of the injured patient begins with the arrival of the ambulance crew and other emergency personnel. They can tell you about the initial condition of the patient and subsequent developments during transfer. Details of the accident itself will enable a more accurate assessment of the severity of injury and likely injuries sustained (see Box 2.1).

Box 2.1 **Factors associated with serious injury:**

• High-speed impact
• Fall from a height of greater than 15 feet
• Death of another person in the same accident
• Entrapment
• Intrusion of the vehicle into the passenger compartment
• Ejection of the patient from the vehicle
• Pedestrian or motorcyclist hit by motor vehicle

Ensure that the emergency crew do not leave the department until this information has been received.

'ABCDE' is a useful *aide-mémoire* for examination and treatment (Box 2.2).

Box 2.2 **The ABC of trauma**

A—airway (with cervical spine control).
B—breathing
C—circulation
D—disability (assessment of neurological deficit)
E—(secondary survey of complete patient)

A—Airway

• **Hypoxia   Oxygenation   Intubation   Ventilation**

Patients will die of hypoxia before they die of hypovolaemia. Signs of hypoxia commonly include pallor, sweating, restlessness, confusion, and agitation; thus the patient pulling off his oxygen mask and pulling out intravenous lines must be recognized as likely to be hypoxic, and not merely uncooperative. Note that cyanosis requires at least 5 g/l of reduced haemoglobin to be present, and is usually absent in hypoxic, hypovolaemic patients.

A pulse oximeter is the cheapest and most effective tool for continuous monitoring of peripheral oxygenation, and can rapidly detect falls in arterial saturation (SaO_2). SaO_2 is normally about 97 per cent when breathing room air, and the reasons for a fall below 95 per cent in a patient must be rapidly identified and corrected. Nevertheless, pulse oximeters do not provide any substitute for the regular and repeated clinical assessment of such patients, and in shocked patients their readings may be misleading. For example, carbon dioxide retention (hypercapnia) can occur in the presence of a normal SaO_2, and pulse oximetry will not detect this. Similarly, the oximeter will not differentiate between carboxyhaemoglobin and oxyhaemoglobin, and may give erroneously high SaO_2 levels in patients with carbon monoxide poisoning.

The airway should be cleared with an initial finger sweep, and mucus, vomit, blood, and other debris should be aspirated with a Yankauer suction catheter. The mouth and oropharynx should be carefully inspected for the presence of foreign bodies, particularly chewing-gum and broken teeth. Partial dental plates or loose-fitting dentures should be removed.

Administer 100 per cent oxygen (10 l/min) initially via a tight-fitting face-mask. Support the neck by applying in-line traction with the hands on the side of the head until a firm cervical collar is securely in place.

Oxygen toxicity is not a problem in the initial resuscitation of trauma patients, and 100 per cent oxygen should be given at least until the patient is stabilized and adequate tissue-oxygenation and arterial blood-gas analysis have been confirmed.

If there is significant damage and/or bleeding in the oropharynx such that the airway is, or may be, compromised, the patient should immediately be given a high concentration of inspired oxygen, and endotracheal intubation considered. This may require the patient to be sedated and given anaesthetic and neuromuscular blocking agents, followed by controlled positive-pressure ventilation (see p. 168). A senior Accident and Emergency specialist with appropriate training or a senior anaesthetist must undertake this. Experience confirms that delays in providing adequate airway procedures until obvious clinical deterioration has occurred compromise future attempts to anaesthetize a progressively hypoxic patient and are associated with increased morbidity and mortality.

Patients who are restless and confused due to hypoxia co-operate poorly with examination and investigation. Their attempts to pull off the oxygen mask or remove intravenous lines increase energy expenditure and aggravate the hypoxic state. The airway-care and anaesthetizing of these patients is particularly difficult, and requires an experienced team approach. Before sedative or neuromuscular blocking drugs are given the patient's neurological status should, where possible, be recorded (see p. 51), provided this will not induce a dangerous delay. Subsequently the patient should be pre-oxygenated with a self-inflating bag and mask with an oxygen reservoir, and a rapid-sequence induction with endotracheal intubation should be performed (see p. 168).

While ideally hypoxia should be confirmed by arterial blood-gas analysis before 'elective' ventilation, attempts to do this must neither delay airway-care nor prolong the hypoxic state. Similarly, where a decision has been made to delay intubation until blood-gas analysis has been performed, these results must be interpreted in the clinical context. Thus, if 'normal' arterial gases are maintained only by administering 100 per cent oxygen, and are associated with tachycardia or tachypnoea, this can only be a temporary state preceding a rapid deterioration. The decision to ventilate such patients should be made sooner rather than later.

B—Breathing

• **Ventilation   Chest injury   Tube thoracostomy**

In general, hypoxic patients do not deteriorate gradually. Decompensation is often rapid and unpredictable.

The diaphragm is the most significant muscle of respiration, and its efficiency is reduced by hypoxia. Increased respiratory effort by the use of the accessory neck and intercostal muscles will fail to achieve oxygen-delivery requirements. As a consequence the respiratory rate increases, and the efforts to maintain respiration become laboured. Passive movement of the now non-functioning diaphragm occurs with caudal movement into the chest during inspiration, depressing vital capacity and leading to a 'hollowed out' appearance of the abdomen. The diaphragm descends into the abdomen during expiration, increasing pulmonary dead space and 'filling out' the abdominal contour. This 'see-saw' movement of chest and abdomen with respiration (so-called paradoxical breathing) indicates diaphragmatic failure, and signals imminent respiratory arrest. Such patients require prompt control of ventilation.

Positive-pressure ventilation reverses the normal physiological consequences of respiration. Reduction in venous return, due to a rise in intrathoracic pressure during 'inspiration', may lead to a fall in cardiac output. This will precipitate circulatory collapse if the circulating blood-volume is already reduced. Additionally, rises in intrathoracic pressure during positive-pressure ventilation increase the risk of pneumothorax in patients with chest injuries, and may induce 'tension' in existing pneumothoraces. This effect must be anticipated, and chest drains must be inserted for *all* patients with pneumothoraces in whom ventilation is to be performed.

The use of anaesthetic and neuromuscular blocking drugs to allow controlled ventilation may mask or modify the clinical features of neurological or abdominal injury. Clearly early and accurate neurological assessment should be performed; but control of the airway and ensuring adequate ventilation must take priority. This may necessitate the use of CT scanning of the head in such patients whenever a head-injury is suspected. Similarly, abdominal injury is notoriously underestimated in patients with altered consciousness due to head-injury, alcohol, or sedation, and further investigations such as diagnostic peritoneal lavage will be required (see p. 86).

When a clear secure airway has been established ensure that ventilation is adequate. Assess chest movement clinically, and auscultate the lung fields to ensure that air enters both lungs normally and symmetrically.

'Sucking' chest wounds should be sealed immediately to prevent further intrathoracic contamination; but objects penetrating the chest should be left undisturbed.

External signs of injury to the chest in a patient continuing to deteriorate despite an established airway, oxygenation, and volume-replacement, must prompt the insertion of a chest drain on the injured side. If the patient's condition fails to improve, repeat the procedure on the other side. To await a chest X-ray before undertaking tube thoracostomy in these circumstances is often a fatal error.

Even in the absence of obvious external signs of injury to the chest, the insertion of bilateral chest drains in obtunded injured patients is indicated if intubation and positive-pressure ventilation have failed to improve their condition.

Clearly this 'aggressive' approach to tube thoracostomy will occasionally lead to the placement of thoracostomy tubes when no pneumothorax is present. If the method of insertion outlined on p. 164 is followed, the risk of misplacement and intrathoracic damage is minimized. The danger in delaying treatment of a tension pneumothorax in a hypoxic hypovolaemic patient is so great that the balance of risk falls in favour of this approach.

If good air-entry is present in both lung fields, and the patient is not deteriorating, a chest radiograph is obtained. The film will be a supine one: fluid levels from haemothoraces will not always be seen, and pneumothoraces can be difficult to identify. An initial 'normal' radiograph does not exclude the later development of a significant lesion, and the need for chest drainage must constantly be considered.

C—Circulation

• **Shock   CVP   IV Access**

Blood-loss and the subsequent reflex compensatory changes contribute to the clinical picture of a patient in shock. The rule is to place 'big drips in big veins', and to restore circulating-volume losses as rapidly as possible. The antecubital fossa veins are often adequate initially, although percutaneous access to the subclavian, jugular, and femoral veins may be required later (see p. 158).

Central venous catheters do not permit adequate flow-rates for rapid volume-replacement, and have no place in the initial stages of resuscitation; although later, when further fluid requirements are being assessed, they may be required.

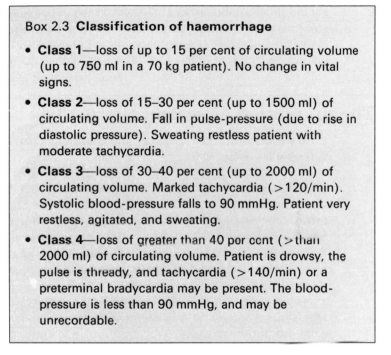

Box 2.3 **Classification of haemorrhage**

- **Class 1**—loss of up to 15 per cent of circulating volume (up to 750 ml in a 70 kg patient). No change in vital signs.

- **Class 2**—loss of 15–30 per cent (up to 1500 ml) of circulating volume. Fall in pulse-pressure (due to rise in diastolic pressure). Sweating restless patient with moderate tachycardia.

- **Class 3**—loss of 30–40 per cent (up to 2000 ml) of circulating volume. Marked tachycardia ($>$120/min). Systolic blood-pressure falls to 90 mmHg. Patient very restless, agitated, and sweating.

- **Class 4**—loss of greater than 40 per cent ($>$than 2000 ml) of circulating volume. Patient is drowsy, the pulse is thready, and tachycardia ($>$140/min) or a preterminal bradycardia may be present. The blood-pressure is less than 90 mmHg, and may be unrecordable.

Box 2.3 illustrates the fact that the 'classical' signs of shock, namely, a fall in blood-pressure and a rise in pulse-rate, are delayed until patients are likely to have lost 30 per cent of their circulating blood-volume. Intravenous volume-replacement must ideally begin before such changes are manifest, so as to minimize the duration of tissue hypoxia. This will go some way to prevent the major consequences of prolonged tissue hypoxia, namely the adult respiratory-distress syndrome and multiple organ-failure.

Major thoracic injuries may require immediate thoracotomy (see Chapter 4), and should be suspected in patients with obvious chest-injuries who have failed to respond to oxygenation, ventilation, tube thoracostomy, and volume-replacement.

D—(Neurological) Deficit

The patient's initial conscious state should be recorded using the Glasgow Coma Scale (see p. 50), and any neurological deficit should be noted. Subsequent changes in the patient's conscious state must be clearly recorded. Any deterioration in conscious state should prompt a re-evaluation of the above ABC factors of airway control, ventilation, and volume-replacement.

The prevention of second 'accidents'

- **Stabilization of cervical spine   Oxygenation   Compound fractures   Pain relief**

All patients involved in high-speed accidents will have subjected their cervical spines to severe acceleration and deceleration forces. Cervical fractures and dislocations are not always painful, and their features may be masked by the pain of other injuries or by alterations in the conscious state of the patient due to primary head-injury, alcohol, or drugs. Patients with altered conscious states also fail to exhibit the protective muscle-spasm which may guard the neck against further movement and injury. Injuries to the head are often also associated with injuries to the cervical spine. For these reasons all patients admitted to the resuscitation room with serious injuries or with an altered conscious state must be assumed to have an unstable neck-injury until proven otherwise.

Hypoxia will exacerbate any cervical cord-injury; and hence the importance of oxygenation, airway-control, and ventilation is paramount. If a cervical spine-injury has been proven or is strongly suspected, endotracheal intubation is not contra-indicated, but requires a highly experienced operator to avoid unnecessary movement of the cervical spine, and hence additional cord-injury. Alternative means of airway control are occasionally required in these patients (see p. 173).

Compound fractures should be covered to prevent further contamination. The use of Polaroid pictures of the wound on arrival, followed by covering with a povidone–iodine soak and a sterile towel or 'clingfilm' is recommended. The wound should not be disturbed subsequently until the time of definitive surgery. Some fractures/dislocations—for example, those of the elbow, knee, and ankle—may threaten the viability of overlying skin or the limb circulation distally. These hazards can be minimized by appropriate manipulation of the limb and reduction of the dislocation, followed by splintage. It is neither necessary nor desirable to achieve perfect anatomical alignment at this stage. Changes in distal pulses and skin perfusion should be clearly noted and recorded before and after such manipulations.

Pain, transmitted by afferent nocioceptive fibres, will increase the sympathoadrenal responses, with catecholamine release leading to increased oxygen-utilization and reduced tissue perfusion. The immediate reduction of gross displacement at fracture sites and careful splintage of long-bone fractures will reduce oxygen demands by limiting pain, and will also reduce the amount of analgesia required.

Analgesia

• **Entonox Opiates Local anaesthesia**

The requirement for analgesia in a patient following injury requires careful and individual consideration. No dogmatic guidelines can be given as to the specific dosage or use of agents required, but the treatment should be tailored to each patient's requirements. With careful and appropriate splintage of long-bone fractures, some patients may require no analgesia at all.

Entonox (50 per cent nitrous oxide, 50 per cent oxygen) is useful for conscious, co-operative patients, and can provide good analgesia, particularly for manipulations or other short, but painful, interventions. However, in patients with altered consciousness, those with airway or ventilation problems, or those in whom chest injuries or pneumothoraces are present, Entonox should not be used.

Intravenous opioids given in small aliquot doses, and carefully titrated to the patient's response, will often be required. The use of a familiar opioid such as Morphine or Diamorphine (preferably with an anti-emetic such as Cyclizine) is recommended. There are no advantages in using the newer (and more expensive) opioid analgesics. Provided that the opioid is titrated in 1–2 mg aliquots given intravenously over 1–2 minutes, problems of overdosage or adverse reactions are rare. Should any untoward actions occur, the effects of the agents described can be reversed completely by Naloxone given intravenously in a dosage of 0.4–1.2 mg.

It should be noted that the presence of a head-injury is not an absolute contraindication to the use of opioid drugs, provided that they are administered in this way and that the patient's airway and ventilation are closely monitored. Whenever these drugs are given, the dose, time, and route of administration must be clearly indicated both on the notes and to the receiving specialist. The use of the specific opioid antagonist Naloxone can also be used where any doubt exists as to whether alterations in a patient's conscious state are due to an administered opioid drug, or related to head-injury and its sequelae.

Local anaesthetic techniques have a limited role in patients with multiple injuries, but nerve-blocks can be valuable for patients with femoral fractures. The procedure is described on p. 166. The use of such a block together with appropriate splintage will minimize the need for additional analgesia, and make the patient more comfortable during the initial phases of management.

Treatments which can commence before definitive diagnosis. The above techniques of oxygenation, cervical spine protection, intubation, ventilation, volume-replacement, tube thoracostomy, and fracture-splintage can and should be performed when indicated and without delay. These procedures and techniques will be performed when the balance of probability, rather than definitive diagnosis, supports their use.

Anti-tetanus prophylaxis and antibiotics for patients with compound skeletal injuries or head-injuries should be administered according to local guidelines.

Radiography and other immediate investigations

While radiological investigation is important in the initial phase of resuscitation, the patient's condition and the ability to continue treatment and monitor the response closely must never be compromised while achieving these investigations.

Fixed (overhead) X-ray facilities within the Resuscitation Room are invaluable, and provide the ability to obtain and rapidly process good-quality radiographs. Where this facility is not possible within the Resuscitation Room, the transfer of an unstable trauma patient to an X-ray room or department leads to unnecessary and often major risk. Therefore, although often of poor quality, initial radiographs should be performed using portable X-ray equipment in the Resuscitation Room.

Box 2.4 Radiographs in the resuscitation room

1. Essential:
- Chest
- Lateral cervical spine (including C1–T1)
- Pelvis

2. Where time and the patient's condition permit:
- Lateral skull
- Lateral thoracic and lumbar spine

Three radiographs are of prime importance:

The first is a chest X-ray. Invariably this will be a supine film, and the limitations of this in the detection of pneumo- or haemothorax and in detecting widening of the mediastinum must be recognized (see p. 75).

A lateral (cross-table) radiograph of the cervical spine (which must include all the vertebrae from C1 to T1) will normally be the second film. It is imperative to know if an unstable neck-injury is present, as it will determine the techniques used in advanced airway-care and in later transportation of the patient. It must however be remembered that injury to the cervical cord can occur with normal radiographic appearances, and movement of the patient and any interventions must be undertaken with this in mind.

Perhaps surprisingly, given the size, shape and nature of the pelvic girdle, clinical detection of pelvic injury is often poor in the early stages of management. External signs of pelvic injury are late to appear, and the technique of 'springing' the pelvis is of little diagnostic value. Since large amounts of blood can be lost from pelvic fractures with little in the way of clinical clues it is important that such patients have an antero-posterior view of the pelvis taken at an early stage. In particular the sacro-iliac regions must be inspected closely, as major disruptions often lead to significant and concealed haemorrhage (see Chapter 6).

Further radiographs, particularly of limbs, should wait until cardiovascular stability has been achieved, and may need to be performed in theatre following laparotomy or thoracotomy. Where time permits however, a lateral skull film and a lateral view of the thoraco-lumbar spine are the most important other radiographic examinations indicated.

During the initial establishment of intravenous access blood will have been taken for cross-matching and other investigations as detailed in Box 2.5. Regular and repeated estimations of arterial blood-gases should be performed, particularly either if these have shown any initial abnormality, such as hypoxaemia or hyper-capnia, or following any intervention to the airway or ventilatory care of the patient.

Box 2.5 Immediate investigations

- Blood Grouping and Cross-matching.
- Arterial Blood gas analysis.
- Haematocrit
- Urea and electrolytes

The roles of diagnostic peritoneal lavage, ultrasound, and CT scanning of the abdomen are outlined in Chapter 5.

Further examination

● Expose patient   Log roll   Rectal examination   Minor injuries

At the earliest possible opportunity following the immediate resuscitative procedures, the patient should be completely exposed and externally examined from head to toe. In particular the back and perineum must be carefully inspected, and this will usually involve log-rolling the patient.

Log-rolling of the patient should be performed with the team-leader taking charge of the patient's airway, head, and neck, and providing gentle, in-line traction while the patient is rolled. During the procedure the patient's nose must stay in line with his navel. Even with a firm collar in place, this manoeuvre can produce antero-posterior movement of the cervical spine, and the doctor must prevent this by gentle traction. With the patient on his side, the spine should then be palpated along its entire length for tenderness and any 'gaps' indicating spine-injury. The external urethral meatus should be examined for blood—suggesting urethral injury. In the male, rectal examination will identify the position of the prostate, which may be displaced upwards or have a boggy sensation following urethral injury. Rectal examination will also detect blood in the rectum, indicating bowel-injury. The anal reflex should be observed, and sensation in the perineum tested and recorded.

During the examination of the entire patient many minor injuries, which may not be life-threatening, but if missed will lead to permanent disability, will be noted, and should be recorded at this stage. Their definitive treatment will often require to be postponed until the more serious conditions have been resolved. Remember that the injuries noted in the Resuscitation Room and on initial radiographic examination are of baseline value, and not definitive. Such patients will require full and regular clinical examination of all the systems over the following few hours and days to detect these more minor and non-life-threatening injuries, which may be masked at the time of initial presentation.

PART 2

System assessment

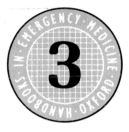

CHAPTER 3

Head-injury

Key points in head-injury

1 A deteriorating conscious level—a fall in the Glasgow Coma Scale is the most significant sign of the development of increased intracranial pressure, and a hallmark of secondary brain-injury.

2 Focal neurological signs usually occur late, and are associated with brain-shifts.

3 Hypovolaemia in the presence of multiple injuries is 'never' due to a head-injury.

4 Hypoxia, hypercapnia, and hypovolaemia must be corrected before the patient is transferred or undergoes CT scanning.

5 When an expanding intracranial haematoma is suspected or diagnosed, endotracheal intubation, sedation, analgesia, and neuromuscular blocking drugs allowing controlled hyperventilation and adequate oxygenation should be considered the rule.

Head-injury: a general introduction

- **Epidemiology** **Primary and secondary brain injuries**

In Great Britain, almost 2000 patients per 100 000 population attend an Accident and Emergency Department annually with head-injury. Of these, between 200 and 400 will require admission, and nine will die. In the context of multiple injury, head-injury accounts for 25 per cent of all deaths.

Injury can occur to the scalp, skull, and brain, independently or in combination. It is damage to the brain, however, that concerns us most, and the association of this with injury to the scalp and skull increases the importance of the early recognition of damage to these structures.

Damage to the brain can occur directly as a result of the original injury (primary brain-damage) or indirectly as a result of other factors (secondary brain-damage). The principal causes of secondary brain-damage are hypoxia, hypovolaemia, increases in intracranial pressure secondary to cerebral oedema or haematoma formation, and cerebral infection. They may arise either as a consequence of the primary brain-injury or of complicating other injuries incurred at the same time.

Clinical assessment

- **Glasgow coma scale** **Neurological history and examination**

The degree, duration, and pattern of conscious level is crucial in the clinical assessment of a head-injured patient. In the past, objective description has been difficult, because words such as 'drowsy' and 'comatose' have different meanings for different doctors. A uniform method of assessing conscious level by scoring levels of responsiveness developed by neurosurgeons in Glasgow addresses this problem, and the Glasgow Coma Scale (GCS) is recognized and used world-wide as a method of measuring conscious state following head-injury (see Fig. 3.1). In addition to providing a common language to describe degrees of coma, the

Glasgow Coma Scale

Eyes	Open	Spontaneously	4
		To verbal command	3
		To pain	2
	No Response		1
Best motor response	To verbal command	Obeys	6
	To painful stimulus*	Localizes pain	5
		Flexion-withdrawal	4
		Flexion-abnormal (Decorticate rigidity)	3
		Extension (Decerebrate rigidity)	2
		No response	1
Best verbal response		Oriented and converses	5
		Disoriented and converses	4
		Inappropiate words	3
		Incomprehensible sounds	2
		No response	1
Total			3-15

Fig. 3.1 • The Glasgow Coma Scale

GCS enables early changes in conscious state to be recognized, and allows intervention to precede irreparable secondary damage. Any change in the GCS with time is particularly important, and the assessment must be performed and recorded regularly. Together with the Glasgow Coma Scale the pupillary sizes and responses to light should be recorded, together with the presence of cerebrospinal fluid (CSF) coming from the ears or nose, any sensory deficit, and the deep tendon reflexes, including the plantar responses.

Box 3.1 Neurological examination

Glasgow Coma Scale

Pupil sizes and responses to light

Examination of ears and nose for blood, CSF haemotympanum

Sensation (including the perianal area)

Deep tendon reflexes (including plantar responses)

Box 3.2 Neurological history

This will be obtained from witnesses, the ambulance crew, or other emergency service personnel.

1. What were the circumstances of the accident? (RTA, speeds involved, falls, etc.)
2. Has the patient talked at any time?
3. What was the patient's Glasgow Coma Score at the accident scene?
4. Has the patient's GCS altered *en route*?
5. Has the patient taken alcohol, or any other drugs?
6. Has the patient had a 'fit'?

Alcohol and head-injury

- **Alcohol and conscious state   Hypoglycaemia**

The ingestion of alcohol can affect the conscious state, and is also associated with an increased chance of sustaining head-injury. However, the relationship between blood- or breath-alcohol levels and conscious state is complex, and varies considerably between individuals. Interpretation of blood- and breath-alcohol levels is fraught with difficulty, and rarely helpful in clinical management. The only safe policy is to note the presence of alcohol, but to ignore its contribution to the clinical state, and to proceed according to the clinical requirements of the patient.

Alcohol can also alter conscious state by inducing hypoglycaemia. Therefore all patients with altered consciousness must have 'stix' testing of capillary blood to detect this, and if it is present correction with intravenous glucose or glucagon must be performed.

Scalp-injury

- **Scalp wounds   Penetrating injuries   Control of haemorrhage**

Haemorrhage from scalp-wounds is often brisk, and occasionally life-threatening, particularly in infants and small children; but adults are also at risk if the wound is large or bleeding is prolonged. Patients with bleeding tendencies, or those on anticoagulant therapy, are at increased risk both from scalp-wounds and from the development of intracranial haematomata.

The scalp-wound should be carefully inspected for foreign bodies, underlying fractures, and herniating brain. The true extent of scalp-injury can only be assessed after the hair has been trimmed and shaved for a centimetre around the edges of the wound. Loose, superficial foreign bodies can be removed; but penetrating or impaled objects should be left undisturbed pending further investigation. Herniation of brain-tissue through the skull table is a poor prognostic indicator. If present, the wound should be covered with a sterile saline-soaked towel, and the advice of a neurosurgeon should immediately be obtained. In the mean time, the resuscitation of the patient continues, as described in Chapter 2.

Scalp-wounds can be probed gently with the finger of a sterile gloved hand to determine the depth of the wound. If the galea has been breached, the likelihood of fracture and underlying brain-injury is high. Fractures are often more easily palpated than visualized, but must be differentiated from the cranial sutures.

Haemorrhage from even the largest scalp-wounds can be controlled by through and through closure of the scalp using interrupted sutures. In the emergency setting, 2/0 or 3/0 silk is easy to handle for this. Additional direct pressure followed by a pressure-dressing may be useful. Otherwise, the wound is covered with non-adherent gauze and secured with a dressing. Haemostasis must be achieved before transfer to a neurosurgical unit, and most scalp-wounds, including those overlying compound fractures, should be closed prior to transport. Debridement of tissue is not usually indicated in the Resuscitation Room. The vascular scalp recovers well from crush-injury, and only obviously grossly damaged tissue should be trimmed during the initial repair.

Skull-fracture

- **Brain damage   Haematomas   CT Scanning   Anaesthesia Neurosurgery   Antibiotic therapy   Basal Skull-fractures Auroscopy   Haemotympanum**

Forces large enough to bruise the scalp may fracture the skull beneath. The relevance of this is that the impact will be transmitted to the underlying brain. The fractured skull may move downwards, leading to a depressed fracture, and either damage brain directly or lead to rupture of underlying blood-vessels, hence damaging the brain indirectly by haematoma formation.

Skull-fracture can however occur with minimal external evidence in the scalp. The close relationship between skull-fracture and intracranial haematoma in adults makes the detection of a fracture important. If there is no skull-fracture on good-quality specimens of the three standard skull radiographs (antero-posterior, lateral, and Towne's views) the risk of intracranial haematoma in a fully conscious—that is, a Glasgow Coma Scale 15/15 patient—is of the order of 0.3 per cent. The presence of a skull-fracture in the same patient increases the risk by a factor of 10, to 3 per cent. If the patient has altered consciousness but no fracture, the risk of haematoma is about 1 per cent; while if the patient is not fully conscious and has a radiologically demonstrable skull-fracture, the risk of developing an intracranial haematoma is as high as 25 per cent.

The discovery of a skull-fracture indicates that a primary brain-injury will have occurred, although the severity of this may still be uncertain, and that secondary brain-injury may occur.

Box 3.3 Guidelines for CT scanning following head-injury

Patients undergoing CT examination *must* have

• a secure airway

• adequate ventilation (controlled where necessary)

• circulating blood-volume deficits corrected

• further haemorrhage—for example, from intra-abdominal or intra-thoracic sites—controlled

All patients must be accompanied by a senior, experienced medical and nursing team together with adequate equipment.

Immediate CT scan

1. Patients in coma—Glasgow Coma Scale 8 or less. (Such patients have a chance of intracranial haematoma of more than 40 per cent.)

2. Patients with depression of conscious level—GCS 9–13—associated with skull-fracture. (The chance of haematoma or other significant intracranial lesions in these patients is approximately 20 per cent.)

3. Patients who deteriorate with a progression to coma (GCS 8 or less).

Urgent CT scan (within six hours)

1. Patients who are drowsy and/or disorientated—GCS 14–15—and have a skull-fracture. (These patients have a chance of intracranial haematoma of 15 per cent.)

2. Patients with abnormal neurological signs together with a skull-fracture.

3. Patients with depression of conscious level (GCS 9–13) together with focal neurological deficit, irrespective of the presence of skull-fracture.

For patients with multiple injuries requiring operative procedures under general anaesthesia, and who are less than 15 on the Glasgow Coma Scale, it is important to exclude positively an intracranial haematoma. These patients should normally undergo CT scanning prior to surgery *provided that the patient's airway, ventilation, and circulation are secure.* If this is not so then the patient should undergo whatever operative intervention—for example, laparotomy/thoracotomy—is required, and have CT scanning immediately following this.

All depressed or compound fractures should be referred to the neurosurgical team for possible elevation and future follow-up. For compound skull-fractures some neurosurgeons advocate prophylactic antibiotic therapy, and the combination of benzyl penicillin (1 mega-unit intravenously) and sulphadimidine (1 g intravenously) is commonly used. Erythromycin or chloramphenicol are alternatives for patients allergic to penicillin. These policies vary considerably on a local basis, and the advice of the neurosurgical team should be sought as to the appropriate agents and indications.

Basal skull-fractures are usually not seen on standard radiographic views of the skull. A basal skull-fracture communicating with a sinus or the middle ear permits air to enter the cranial vault, and this may be seen on a skull radiograph. It is easiest to recognize on a lateral skull film viewed in the position in which it was taken, with the brow up. A black line of air will be seen at the uppermost point, adjacent to the inner skull table. The diagnosis of basal skull-fracture is, however, made largely on clinical grounds, although CT scanning can be helpful. A patient with altered consciousness or evidence of head-injury and with bleeding from the ear should be considered to have a middle-fossa basal skull-fracture until it is proven otherwise. Where bleeding from the ear is present auroscopy may introduce infection, and is rarely helpful. Where bleeding is not present, however, it is important to exclude haemotympanum.

It is rare to see pure cerebrospinal fluid from the ear or nose in the early stages following injury, and testing for the glucose content of any secretion is unhelpful. Bleeding from the nose in the absence of local injury must be assumed to be due to a fracture of the floor of the frontal fossa, and hence the insertion of a nasogastric tube is contraindicated.

Because of the fact that basal skull-fractures may communicate with the sinuses and/or middle ear, these injuries are compound in nature. The risk of intracranial infection is high, and prophylactive antibiotic as detailed above should be considered. Basal fractures associated with severe facial fractures pose major practical difficulties. Their early recognition is essential. The immediate life-threatening problem is the often torrential blood-flow from the facial skeleton into the posterior oropharynx, leading to pulmonary aspiration. Even if aspiration does not occur, the magnitude of haemorrhage can produce hypovolaemic shock. LeFort III fractures with facial mobility can be 'reduced' by pulling on the maxilla until the face fills out. This can reduce haemorrhage, but is extremely painful, and should only be considered in anaesthetized or deeply unconscious patients. Facio-maxillary surgeons must be involved as soon as possible, and in conjunction with the neurosurgical team will determine further steps towards haemostasis.

Brain-injury

• **Features of primary brain damage   Causes and prevention of secondary brain damage   Use of drugs   Intracranial haematomata**

Primary brain-damage occurs as a result of the initial injury, rather than as a consequence of subsequent or coincidental events. It can be due to direct-impact damage from blunt or penetrating injury and/or a result of rotational forces and contre-coup injuries induced by the impact.

Movement of the brain after impact causes surface shear lesions, and produces contusions of the brain-matter, particularly in the frontal or temporal regions. Intracerebral haematomata, subarachnoid haemorrhage, and brain lacerations may occur as a direct consequence of the impact, or as the brain moves quickly over the irregular surface of the cranial floor. Diffuse white-matter injury can also occur primarily; but its devastating effects are usually only of practical relevance to the pathologist!

The degree of primary brain-damage correlates with the period of altered consciousness and post-traumatic amnesia. Whenever a history of loss of consciousness is present, diffuse brain-injury has occurred. The patient's return to full consciousness may be rapid, but later questioning often reveals that new memory was not laid down for some time after apparent clinical recovery. The primary injury will have produced its effects prior to hospital arrival. The primary role of the trauma team is to prevent further deterioration, by recognizing and correcting those factors producing secondary brain-damage.

A deteriorating conscious level—a fall in Glasgow Coma Scale—with or without localizing neurological signs is the hallmark of progressive secondary brain-injury. The commonest cause of this is hypoxia. The patient's airway, ventilation, and circulation must always be reassessed, and where appropriate corrected, before CT scanning or other intervention. Hypoxia leads to a fall in cerebral energy metabolism, a rise in intracranial pressure (ICP), cerebral oedema, and eventually cerebral coning and death.

Hypovolaemia, often concurrent with hypoxia, also commonly leads to secondary brain-injury. The importance of maintaining cardiac output and adequate cerebral perfusion in head-injury cannot be overemphasized, particularly when injuries to the head form only part of the complex picture of multiple injury. Although exsanguinating open brain-injuries can occur, for all practical purposes it is imperative that hypotension in the presence of head-injury is assumed to be secondary to haemorrhage from other (often unrecognized) injuries. Most frequently, this is related to intraperitoneal or intrathoracic blood-loss.

Alone or in combination, hypoxia, hypercapnia, poor cerebral perfusion, and cerebral contusion are among the factors that may lead to raised intracranial pressure (see Box 3.4). The importance of recognizing changes in ICP are that they may reflect these secondary insults. A rise in intracranial pressure leads to convolutional flattening, followed by herniation of the brain

NEUROLOGICAL OBSERVATION CHART

NAME   UNIT No
                    D. of B.
                    WARD

DATE   TIME

C O M A	Eyes open	Spontaneously	4	Eyes closed by swelling =C
		To speech	3	
		To pain	2	
		None	1	
	Best verbal response	Orientated	5	Endotrachea tube or Tracheostomy =T
		Confused	4	
		Inappropriate Words	3	
		Incomprehensible Sounds	2	
		None	1	
S C A L E	Best motor response	Obey commands	6	Usually records the best arm response
		Localise pain	5	
		Normal Flexion	4	
		Abnormal Flexion	3	
		Extension to pain	2	
		None	1	

COMA SCALE TOTAL 3 — 15

INTRACRANIAL PRESSURE

Pupil scale (m.m.)
• 1
• 2
• 3
● 4
● 5
● 6
● 7
● 8

240
230
220
210
200
190
180
170
160
150
140
130
120
110
100
90
80
70
60
50
Respiration 40
30
26
22
18
14
10
6

40
39
38 Temperature °C
37
36
35
34
33
32
31
30

PUPILS	right	Size		+ reacts
		Reaction		− no reaction
	left	Size		c. eye closed
		Reaction		

L I M B	A R M S	Normal power		Record right (R) and left (L) separately if there is a difference between the two sides.
		Mild weakness		
		Severe weakness		
		Extension		
		No response		
M O V E M E N T	L E G S	Normal power		
		Mild weakness		
		Severe weakness		
		Extension		
		No response		

Fig. 3.2 • A neurological observation chart

around the brain-stem, with distortion, haemorrhage, and infarction. When herniation occurs centrally through the tentorium, brain-stem buckling, distortion, and loss of blood-supply occurs. This is accompanied by venous obstruction and ischaemic infarction in the mid-brain. The patient is unresponsive, with small pupils and 'doll's eye' movements, and symmetrical long-tract signs are present.

Cerebral blood-flow, and hence cerebral perfusion, is determined by the gradient between mean arterial pressure and mean intracranial pressure. Any reduction in cerebral perfusion will itself increase intracranial pressure, leading to the establishment of a vicious circle. Thus the correction and prevention of the factors in Box 3.4 are paramount in prevention of secondary brain-injury.

Box 3.4 Factors increasing intracranial pressure

1. Hypoxia
2. Hypercapnia
3. Hypotension
4. Intracranial haemorrhage
5. Intracranial infection

Rapid increases in intracranial pressure associated with cerebral oedema or an expanding haematoma may present as a fit. The patient who has a fit following a head-injury should have the seizure controlled with intravenous diazepam or phenytoin, together with appropriate airway-control and ventilation.

To prevent, or minimize, rises in ICP, PaO_2 levels should be maintained between 15 and 20 kPa. Hypercapnia causes cerebral vasodilation, and hence increases intracranial pressure. The control and prevention of hypercapnia and the maintenance of a $PaCO_2$ at 3.5–4.0 kPa will prevent this. Further reductions in $PaCO_2$ are unhelpful, and may lead to cerebral vasoconstriction and reduce oxygen-delivery.

There is no evidence that the administration of steroids or barbiturates significantly reduces intracranial pressure or leads to an improved outcome for head-injury patients. A 20 per cent solution of Mannitol in a dosage of 0.5–1.0 g/kg body weight intravenously over 15–20 minutes may control increased intracranial pressure temporarily by leading to brain-shrinkage. This should not normally be given except under the direct advice of the neurosurgical receiving team, and at best provides a short-lived improvement in intracranial pressure.

Intracranial haematomata

In the context of multiple injury, intracranial haematoma must be suspected when coma persists or develops in spite of adequate airway-control and oxygenation and appropriate fluid-replacement for other injuries. Clinical differentiation of the various types of intracranial haematoma is rarely possible, and of little practical benefit in the initial resuscitative procedure.

The so-called 'classical' signs of an expanding intracranial haematoma (dilated pupil on the side of the lesion, and contralateral hemiparesis) are late and inconsistant signs, and represent established brain-injury. The most significant clinical finding will be a deterioration in conscious level. Any such change must prompt a re-evaluation of the resuscitation priorities in the

---

Box 3.5 **Intracranial haematomata**

1. Extradural—usually related to bleeding from middle meningeal vessels in the temporal or temperoparietal regions

2. Intradural
   a. Subdural—usually due to bleeding from superficial veins ruptured indirectly by shearing forces or directly by impact
   b. Intracerebral—most commonly occurring in the frontal and temporal lobes, and usually associated with immediate impairment of consciousness as a result of associated diffuse white-matter injury

3. Subarachnoid haemorrhage

4. Mixed types

patient, neurosurgical consultation, CT scanning, and, where appropriate, surgery.

In Great Britain it can rarely, if ever, be justified for a non-specialist to execute exploratory burr holes, and, except in extreme circumstances, patients requiring neurosurgical intervention can be transferred to the nearest neurosurgical unit.

Further reading

Gentleman, D. and Jennett, B. (1981). Hazards of interhospital transfer of comatose head injured patients. *Lancet*, **ii**, 853–5.

Grossman, R. G. and Gildenberg, P. L. (ed.) (1982). *Head injury*. Raven Press, New York.

Jennett, B. and Teasdale, G. (1981). *Management of head injury*. F. A. Davis, Philadelphia.

Jennett, B. and McMillan, R. (1981). Epidemiology of head injury. *British Medical Journal*, **282**, 101–4.

Mendelow, A. D. (1990). Management of head injury. *Hospital Update*, **March 1990**, 195–206.

Mendelow, A. D., Teasdale, G., Jennett, B., *et al.* (1983). Risks of intracranial haematoma in head injured adults. *British Medical Journal*, **287**, 1173–6.

Miller, J. D. (1989). Significance and management of intracranial hypertension after head injury, in *Update in intensive care and emergency medicine* ((ed. J. L. Vincent) **8**, 496–501. Springer-Verlag, Berlin.

Miller, J. D., Butterworth, J. F., and Gudeman, S. K. (1981). Further experience in the management of severe head injury. *Journal of Neurosurgery*, **54**, 289–99.

Skull X-ray examinations after head trauma (recommendations by multi-disciplinary panel and validation study) (1987). *New England Journal of Medicine*, **316**, 84–91.

Suggestions from a group of neurosurgeons (1984). Guidelines for initial management after head injury in adults. *British Medical Journal*, **288**, 983–5.

injured, neurosurgical consultation, CT scanning, and, where appropriate, surgery.

Further reading

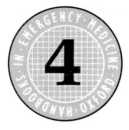

CHAPTER 4

Thoracic injury

Key points in chest-injuries

1 The majority of injuries to the chest can be managed appropriately with oxygenation, intravenous fluid replacement, and tube thoracostomy for haemothorax and pneumothorax. Patients who do not respond to these measures may require intubation and positive-pressure ventilation, and a small proportion may require emergency or urgent thoracotomy.

2 Pneumothoraces secondary to trauma should be drained by means of formal tube thoracostomy. This is mandatory if patients will subsequently have positive-pressure ventilation.

3 For patients with deceleration injuries, and blunt injuries to the chest it is essential to have a high index of suspicion as to the possibility of myocardial and/or major-vessel injury.

Thoracic injury: a general introduction

- Ventilation–perfusion mismatch   Hypovolaemia   Mechanical obstruction

The heart and lungs are neither physiologically nor anatomically separate organs. Together the heart/lung organ oxygenates and circulates the blood as a continuous, integrated process. An injury to either will therefore affect the other, and injuries to both are often devastating.

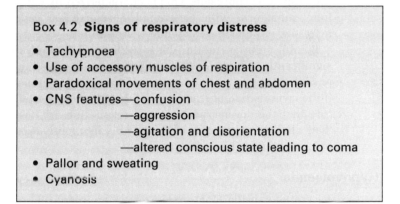

Box 4.2 **Signs of respiratory distress**

- Tachypnoea
- Use of accessory muscles of respiration
- Paradoxical movements of chest and abdomen
- CNS features—confusion
     —aggression
     —agitation and disorientation
     —altered conscious state leading to coma
- Pallor and sweating
- Cyanosis

Chest injuries are the primary cause of death in at least 25 per cent of fatal trauma cases, and contribute to 50 per cent of the remainder. Paradoxically, death is rarely due to failure to perform complex surgery, and overall less than 10–15 per cent of chest trauma cases require formal surgical intervention. The remainder can be managed adequately with a combination of oxygen therapy, intravenous volume-replacement, tube thoracostomy, and controlled ventilation. Much of the terrible death-toll related to chest-injuries is therefore potentially avoidable, or at the least could be reduced by simple standard resuscitative techniques. Despite this, it has been shown that these measures are often not applied, or are performed too late, because the severity and nature of the injury was missed or underestimated. In particular, the physiological impact of injuries such as traumatic pneumothorax cannot be estimated from radiographic appearances alone.

There are several pathophysiological elements to chest-injury:

Ventilation–perfusion mismatch

Ventilation–perfusion mismatch occurs when non-ventilated lung is perfused and intrapulmonary shunting occurs. It is important to note that increasing the inspired oxygen concentration will only increase arterial oxygenation via ventilated areas of lung. Thus even a small degree of shunting and mismatch will significantly reduce the effect of increased inspired oxygen, and result in persistent arterial hypoxaemia. Pulmonary aspiration, inhalation burns, and simple pneumothorax commonly result in ventilation–perfusion mismatch; but the commonest trauma-related cause is probably lung contusion. This is characterized by damage to the lung substance, with associated haemorrhage, oedema, and increases in pulmonary capillary permeability.

Painful injuries to the chest wall inhibit respiration, and significantly reduce tidal volume for a considerable time. Sternal or rib fractures can lead to hypoxia if this effect is pronounced, or if the combination of fractures so disrupts the skeletal architecture that the normal mechanics of respiration are destroyed. A 'flail' chest is an example of this, and is frequently accompanied by contusion of the underlying lung.

Hypovolaemia

Lacerations of the lung or injuries to the intercostal or internal mammary vessels commonly produce significant bleeding and haemothorax. Bleeding from lacerations to the lung parenchyma alone involves low-pressure vessels, and is commonly self-limiting. Injury to the intercostal or internal mammary arteries involves higher pressures, and may not be self-limiting, leading to large haemothoraces; while injury to the great vessels is often fatal.

Mechanical obstruction

Tension pneumothorax and cardiac tamponade are the most serious conditions which reduce cardiac output by preventing adequate cardiac filling. Expanding haematomata within the mediastinum can also compress the venae cavae, preventing venous return to the heart and reducing cardiac output.

Penetrating chest-trauma can produce a single type of injury as outlined above, while blunt chest-trauma more often involves a mixture of the different types. The relative importance of each form of injury may change over time, and may affect other injuries elsewhere.

Thoracic cage injuries

• **Rib fractures**   **Associated injuries**   **Sternal fractures**

The recognition of rib-fractures is important for several reasons. The presence of rib-fractures is an index of the forces involved in the injury, and indicates that underlying structures may also be damaged. Lung contusion or laceration, pneumothorax, and haemothorax may all accompany rib-fractures. In younger patients, the compliance of the chest wall is such that significant compressive forces can be accommodated by the elasticity of the ribs without fracture. However, the underlying lung will still have been compressed and damaged. Compressive force to the chest may disarticulate the costochondral junctions, and alter the mechanics of respiration in the same way as a fracture. In the elderly, the rigid and brittle ribs fracture readily, leading to further injury to the underlying lung.

The upper ribs are normally well-protected by the shoulder complex of clavicle, scapula, and upper limb. Fractures of the first three ribs therefore indicate that considerable force has been involved. Fractures of these ribs are commonly associated with injuries to the aorta and other great vessels, the major bronchi, the brachial plexus, and the heart.

The association of fractures of the ninth, tenth, and eleventh ribs with injuries to the liver and spleen is also well-recognized.

In conscious co-operative patients the diagnosis of injuries to the chest wall is relatively easy, with local tenderness and bony crepitus usually detectable. The presence of surgical emphysema should also alert the clinician to underlying lung or bronchial injury in patients with blunt injuries.

Radiographic assessment of rib-fractures is notoriously inaccurate, with up to 50 per cent of rib-fractures missed on initial radiographs.

Sternal fractures are usually caused by direct blunt injury, and are most often the result of car-drivers striking against their steering-wheels or decelerating suddenly against the diagonal component of their seat-belts. These fractures are transverse, and cause considerable pain. They are best visualized radiographically on a lateral sternal view. However, the prime importance of the injury is the frequent association with blunt injuries to the heart and mediastinum. Sternal fractures may also form one component of a flail segment.

Flail chest

• Definition Recognition Pathological effects

The diagnosis of a flail segment is a clinical one. The involved segment moves (paradoxically) inwards during inspiration and outwards during expiration. The condition occurs when three or more adjacent ribs are fractured at two or more points, with the result that the involved segment can move independently of the remaining chest wall.

The condition is commonly missed; but its recognition is important, as associated underlying lung-injury is common. Initially, splinting of the flail segment by muscle-spasm may make it difficult to see the paradoxical movement. As the muscle-spasm wears off, and lung function deteriorates, the degree of paradoxical movement often becomes more apparent, particularly if the observer's line of sight is in the plane of the chest wall and tangential lighting is used.

The physiological effect of the flail segment is to compromise ventilation by reducing tidal volume and compressing the lung parenchyma beneath the affected area. Hypoventilation, hypoxaemia, intrapulmonary shunting, and reduction in cardiac output follow.

A small flail segment alone does not necessitate mechanical ventilation. Provided the patient's general condition remains stable and regular arterial blood-gas analysis indicates appropriate gas-exchange, such patients may be managed with careful observation, together with high concentrations of inspired oxygen, analgesia, and other appropriate measures. While the use of local analgesia with intercostal nerve-blocks can be helpful, this technique is not recommended in the Emergency Department, but may be applicable in the more controlled environment of the general or thoracic surgical ward, or intensive care unit.

Pneumothorax

- **Definition   Tension pneumothorax   Clinical and radiological detection   Open pneumothorax   Management**

Air accumulates in the potential space between the visceral and parietal pleura in almost all patients with penetrating chest-injuries, and in up to 50 per cent of patients with blunt chest-injuries. After blunt thoracic trauma, pneumothorax is most often related to rib-fractures.

A tension pneumothorax occurs when air collects progressively under pressure in the pleural space as a consequence of a 'flap-valve' mechanism in the underlying injured lung. Air then enters the pleural space during inspiration, and is unable to leave during expiration. As the intrapleural pressure increases, the lung collapses, the mediastinum is deviated to the contralateral side, and the thin-walled vena cava is easily compressed, often with sudden and dramatic reductions in cardiac filling and output. In patients who are already hypoxic and/or hypovolaemic from other injuries even a small degree of 'tension' in a pneumothorax can be catastrophic.

The detection of pneumothorax can be difficult both clinically and radiologically. In the busy hubbub of the Resuscitation Room reduced breath-sounds and hyper-resonance on percussion are often missed. Supine chest radiographs may fail to show the extrapleural air in small pneumothoraces, which may not extend far enough to separate the lung edge from the chest wall at the apex or lateral aspects. Accordingly, where possible, inspiratory and expiratory *erect* chest films should be obtained. It should be emphasized that radiographic confirmation of suspected *tension* pneumothorax is contraindicated. If the diagnosis is clinically suspected then *immediate* needle thoracostomy (p. 163) should be performed to decompress the high intrapleural pressure and allow time for a formal tube thoracostomy to be performed.

Tension pneumothorax is a particular hazard for patients with chest-injuries who are undergoing assisted ventilation. Commonly such patients are sedated, and have received neuromuscular blocking agents; as a consequence the classical clinical features may be missed. A rise in airway-pressure, hypotension, and elevated central venous pressure will occur; and, if untreated, the tension pneumothorax will lead to cardiac arrest.

It is our practice that patients with crush-injuries to the chest, or those with even small traumatic pneumothoraces, should have these drained before positive-pressure ventilation is performed, because of the high risk of developing a tension pneumothorax. The technique for tube thoracostomy is detailed on p. 164.

Open pneumothorax

So-called 'sucking' chest-wounds are exceedingly rare in civilian practice in the United Kingdom, and are usually related to shotgun injuries or impalement. Because the thoracic cage has been breached, intrapleural pressure remains the same as atmospheric pressure, and the ipsilateral lung is unable to expand normally during inspiration.

Sucking chest-wounds should be covered with a sterile occlusive dressing, and formal tube thoracostomy should be performed. Endotracheal intubation and positive-pressure ventilation are often needed in such patients, and provided tube thoracostomy has been performed the pneumothorax will not re-accumulate unless major tracheal or bronchial disruption has occurred.

Haemothorax

- **Association with rib fractures   Radiological aspects Management**

Bleeding into the chest is often associated with pneumothorax. However, even alone the development of a haemothorax increases intrathoracic pressure and leads to collapse of the ipsilateral lung, and thus aggravates the effects of hypovolaemia by reducing cardiac filling and output.

If blood is allowed to clot and organize within the pleural space it will further inhibit lung function, and act as a focus of infection. The clinical diagnosis of haemothorax is often difficult, although its presence may be suspected from already recognized chest-injuries. It is estimated that even a single rib-fracture is associated with the loss of 150 ml of blood into the pleural cavity.

The rate of bleeding into the chest cannot be accurately assessed from clinical examination, nor from chest radiographs. It takes several hundred millilitres of blood to blunt the costophrenic angle, even on an erect chest radiograph. By the time a clear fluid-level is seen across the lung field, several litres may have been lost. The recognition of a haemothorax is even more difficult on supine films, since very large amounts of blood in the pleural space may show no abnormality, or at best only diffuse shadowing of the lung fields. The insertion of a chest drain will enable accurate and continuous assessment of blood-loss and treat any concomitant pneumothorax, which is often masked by the haemothorax. In some units auto-transfusion of blood from haemothoraces has been employed.

Injuries to the heart

- **Myocardial contusion   Septal and valve rupture   Penetrating cardiac injury   Cardiac tamponade   Resuscitation room thoracotomy**

Blunt injury to the chest through rapid deceleration may produce myocardial contusion. This is most often seen following road-traffic accidents, where the restraining action of seat-belts and/or contact with the steering-wheel are the usual events. Fractures of the sternum are the commonest associated bony injury. Damage to the myocardium may produce ECG changes, which range from non-specific ST-T wave changes (often in the anterior chest leads) to the full-blown picture of myocardial infarction. Rhythm disturbances, such as ventricular extra-systoles, and atrial dysrhythmias such as atrial flutter or fibrillation, may result from blunt injury to the conducting system of the heart. Unfortunately, the presence of ECG changes is not invariable, and may take some time to develop. This applies equally to the other commonly used test, where rises in cardiac-specific muscle-enzymes (CPK-MB) are sought.

The history of injury should be the chief indicator as to the possibility of myocardial injury in patients with blunt trauma. The vulnerability of the right ventricle, as a thin-walled structure lying close behind the sternum, is well-recognized, and must be appreciated in all such patients, particularly in those with associated sternal fracture. More severe blunt injury to the heart may result in myocardial rupture (usually involving the ventricles) or rupture of the ventricular septum or valves. Myocardial rupture is rarely associated with survival for long enough to reach hospital; but in those few patients surviving to admission to the Emergency Department the features are those of rapidly developing cardiac tamponade. Patients with septal or valvular ruptures may have the diagnosis missed in the Emergency Department if coexistent hypovolaemia is associated with low-flow states through the heart, and thrills and murmurs are therefore of low intensity. The aortic valve is the most commonly affected, although mitral and tricuspid valve-injury has been reported. Where appropriate, ECG, echo-cardiographic, and cardiac catheterization procedures are indicated.

Penetrating cardiac wound and cardiac tamponade

Penetrating injuries to the heart require immediate diagnosis and intervention. In Great Britain gunshot wounds are very rare; but the frequency of stab wounds to the chest and upper abdomen is increasing dramatically. The direction of such wounds is often difficult to ascertain; but the presence of a wound in the precordial or epigastric region must be a strong pointer as to the possibility of underlying cardiac injury. One should bear in mind that any penetrating wound to the thorax or upper abdomen may involve the heart or mediastinum.

For penetrating wounds involving the heart the right ventricle is most commonly injured, and its thin-walled structure can allow continued bleeding in the absence of tamponade. The left ventricle is the next most commonly injured structure; but its thicker wall can often close off a wound-defect for a time.

The clinical signs of traumatic cardiac tamponade, the so-called Beck's triad of muffled heart-sounds, distended neck veins, and

---

Box 4.1 Clinical features of cardiac tamponade

- Hypotension
- Tachycardia
- Distended neck veins
- Elevated central venous pressure (N.B. C.V.P. may be low or normal in hypovolaemic patients)

Features occasionally seen, but not diagnostic:
- Muffled heart sounds
- Pulsus paradoxus
- Electrical alternans on ECG

---

hypotension, are rarely seen. Changes on ECG are uncommon, and rarely pathognomonic. Chest X-ray may reveal an associated pneumo- or haemothorax; but the cardiac silhouette is frequently normal in patients subsequently proved to have pericardial tamponade. The pericardium is a fibrous and relatively inelastic sack, so that increases in its size and shape rarely occur in the context of acute tamponade.

The presence of an elevated central venous pressure (usually of 15–20 cm), together with associated hypotension and tachycardia, are the most reliable signs of cardiac tamponade. When these are present, and provided a tension pneumothorax has been excluded, then cardiac tamponade should be strongly suspected. In some situations where other injuries have led to hypovolaemia or the pericardium has been able to decompress spontaneously, the central venous pressure may be low or normal. However, a response to volume-replacement by a rise in central venous pressure together with continued hypotension and tachycardia should strongly suggest that cardiac tamponade is present.

If time and the patient's condition permit, echocardiography will provide confirmation of the diagnosis; but this is rarely immediately available in our resuscitation rooms.

One approach to the management of patients with penetrating wound to the chest or abdomen that may have involved the thoracic cavity or heart is outlined (see Fig. 4.1).

In our experience attempts at needle pericardiocentesis are fruitless and lead to delay. In patients with cardiac arrest open

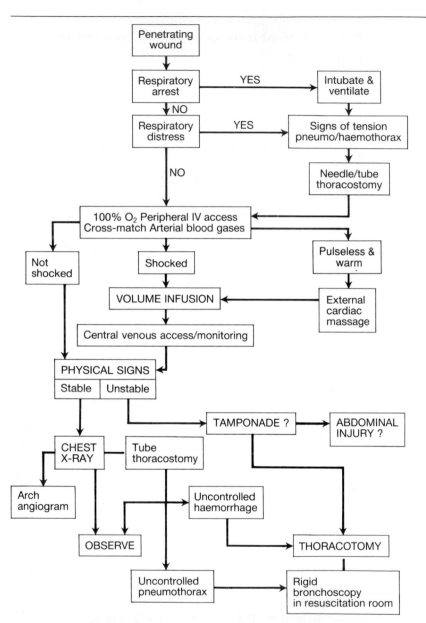

Fig. 4.1 • An algorithm for the management of wounds that may have penetrated the thoracic cavity

thoracotomy (see p. 174) should be performed in the Resuscitation Room. Stable or shocked patients should normally have the procedure performed in a surgical theatre by a thoracic surgical team, provided this can be achieved immediately.

In some studies up to 40 per cent of patients with penetrating wounds to the heart have survived. In general, knife-wounds carry a much better prognosis than gunshot-wounds, owing to the lower velocity and the lesser degree of tissue-destruction involved. Even for patients apparently dead with penetrating injury, up to 30 per cent may survive. Invariably, survival is the result of a prompt recognition of the problem and immediate surgery.

In some centres resuscitation-room thoracotomy has been advocated for patients with cardiac arrest following blunt injury; but in our experience survival is extremely rare, and requires the ability to achieve aortic cross-clamping and cardio-pulmonary bypass.

Aortic injuries

• **Mechanism of injury   Recognition   Radiological features**

Blunt injury to the chest, associated with severe deceleration forces, will lead to damage in those areas where the motion of the internal organs is greatest. The normal cardiac ejection fraction is accommodated by rhythmic motion of the aorta, and this requires some areas to be less tethered to surrounding structures than others. Deceleration forces disrupt the tissue layers of the aorta in these areas, producing localized dissection. The intima is always involved, and often part of the media layer also. The root of the ascending aorta and the descending aorta between the origin of the left subclavian artery and the fourth intercostal artery are the two most vulnerable areas. The former is often associated with acute cardiac tamponade, and accordingly has an even greater mortality.

Overall 80–90 per cent of patients with aortic rupture die within ten minutes of the injury. For patients surviving to reach hospital, injuries to the descending aorta are three times as

Box 4.3 **Commonly seen features on chest radiograph suggesting aortic rupture**

• Widened upper mediastinum
• Trachea deviated to right
• Haemothorax (especially left-sided)
• Blurring of aortic knuckle-shadow
• Deviation of nasogastric tube to right
• Depression of left main bronchus

common as those of the ascending aorta. Rapid diagnosis is dependent upon the recognition of the forces involved and of the possibility of the injury occurring. The presence of severe coexistent injuries to the chest, head, and neck may initially mask the presentation, but should be taken as pointers to the severe forces involved.

Occasionally the presentation may be of paraplegia in the absence of overt spinal injury, or of paradoxical reflex hypertension. A good quality antero-posterior chest X-ray is important for diagnosis. Widening of the mediastinal shadow is not invariable, but is seen in the majority of aortic ruptures. Other associated radiographic features include the presence of a left haemothorax, depression of the left main bronchus, deviation of a nasogastric tube to the right, and loss of the normal aortic knob-shadow. Associated injuries, such as fractures to the first and second ribs or clavicles, may also be identified, although some studies have failed to indicate a significant association between aortic injuries and isolated fractures of the first or second ribs.

We recommend the North American approach to suspected aortic injuries, with the early use of arch aortography, provided that the patient's other injuries permit. Facilities for this in the United Kingdom are considerably more limited, both in terms of expertise and in terms of the availability of this technique; and the use of ultrasound and CT scanning has been advocated. As with penetrating cardiac injuries, there is no place for conservative management of traumatic aortic injury, and a high index of suspicion, together with an aggressive and appropriate approach to thoracic surgical intervention, is essential if these patients are to survive.

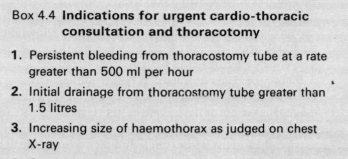

Box 4.4 Indications for urgent cardio-thoracic consultation and thoracotomy

1. Persistent bleeding from thoracostomy tube at a rate greater than 500 ml per hour
2. Initial drainage from thoracostomy tube greater than 1.5 litres
3. Increasing size of haemothorax as judged on chest X-ray
4. Cardiac tamponade or evidence of rupture to the trachea or bronchial tree

Injuries to the lung

- Pulmonary contusion   Fat embolism   ARDS   Bronchial rupture   Oesophageal injury

Compressive forces applied across the chest, either during rapid deceleration or through a direct blow, create capillary and alveolar wall disruption, leading to interstitial and intra-alveolar haemorrhage and oedema. The effects of these changes on pulmonary function may take up to forty-eight hours to develop, and the result is one of progressive intrapulmonary shunting, with hypoxaemia. Ventilation is often required where patients have sustained compressive injury of such a nature that it affects large areas of lung or is found in association with other injuries. Coincidental long-bone fractures, which may be associated with fat emboli, increase the risk of the development of the adult respiratory-distress syndrome, and also the need to provide assisted ventilation to maintain adequate tissue oxygenation.

Of injuries to the tracheal bronchial tree, 80 per cent occur within 1 inch of the carina. Complete transections are usually rapidly fatal; but in some cases local compression by associated injuries delays the development of full rupture. Air-leaks from the tracheo-bronchial tree are associated with the development of pneumomediastinum. This may be seen radiologically, and is occasionally associated with a 'crunching' sound during cardiac

systole (Hamman's sign). Tracking of the air, with the development of subcutaneous emphysema in the neck, head, and
clavipectoral regions, often occurs. In some situations tension
pneumothorax or even tension pneumopericardium can occur.
These features may occur with injuries affecting the oesophagus.
Blunt oesophageal injury is very rare; but penetrating trauma is
more commonly associated with oesophageal injury. Delay in
diagnosis significantly increases the mortality, because of the
development of mediastinitis. Leakage of oesophageal contents
may produce signs in the lungs, and occasionally the diagnosis is
made by leakage of content via a tube thorocostomy. A chest
radiograph may show a nasogastric tube entering the pleural
space, or saliva and gastric contents may drain from a thoracostomy tube. The diagnosis can be confirmed by endoscopy or
contrast radiography. The type of contrast used is somewhat
controversial, as while Gastrographin is less irritant to the lungs
in the event of leakage, it is more damaging if aspirated, and
provides a less sensitive test than standard barium techniques.
Diaphragmatic injuries are outlined on p. 90.

Further reading

Bancewicz, J. and Yates, D. (1983). Blunt injury to the heart. *British
Medical Journal*, **286**, 497.

Berg, G. A., Kirk, A. J. B., and Reece, I. J. (1987). Management of
penetrating chest wounds. *Hospital Update*, November, 949–61.

Bryan, A. J., and Angelini, G. D. (1989). Traumatic rupture of the thoracic
aorta. *British Journal of Hospital Medicine*, **41**, 320–6.

Buckman, R., Trooszkin, S. Z., Flancbaum, L., and Chander, J. (1987). The
significance of stable patients with sternal fracture. *Surgery,
Gynaecology and Obstetrics*, **164**, 261–5.

Mattox, K. L. and Allen, M. K. (1986). Systematic approach to
pneumothorax, haemothorax, pneumomediastinum and subcutaneous emphysema. *Injury*, **17**, 309–12.

Poole, G. V. (1989). Fractures to the upper ribs and injury to the great
vessels. *Surgery, Gynaecology and Obstetrics*, **169**, 275–82.

Taggart, D. P. and Reece, I. J. (1987). Penetrating cardiac injuries
[editorial]. *British Medical Journal*, **294**, 1630–1.

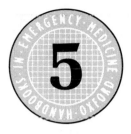

CHAPTER 5

Abdominal injury

Key points in abdominal injury

1 Clinical assessment of the injured abdomen is very unreliable.

2 The recognition that emergency laparotomy is required for abdominal injury is more important than detailed preoperative investigation of the organ (organs) involved.

3 Remember that penetrating injuries to the lower thoracic area (up to the level of the nipple) may traverse the diaphragm, and involve the intra-abdominal contents, and vice versa.

4 Blood tests and plain radiological investigations are in general of little help in the assessment or localization of injury.

5 Diagnostic peritoneal lavage is the single most useful adjunct, but has clearly defined indications and contraindications. Ultrasound/CT scanning may be of value in selected *stable* patients.

6 A naso- or oro-gastric tube should be passed to aspirate stomach contents and relieve gastric dilation. Provided there is no contraindication, a urinary catheter should be inserted to drain the bladder, to detect haematuria, and to enable monitoring of urine output.

7 In patients with blood at the urethral meatus an anterior retrograde urethrogram should be performed before inserting a urinary catheter.

8 The detection of frank haematuria is an indication of significant urinary-tract injury, which, if the patient's condition permits, will require further radiographic assessment by means of intravenous urethrogram and cystogram, and, if necessary, CT scan and/or angiography.

Abdominal injury: a general introduction

* Mechanisms of injury   Blunt vs penetrating trauma

Although rarely as dramatic in presentation, or as immediately life-threatening, as airway or thoracic injury, abdominal trauma is frequently underestimated and poorly managed in the Emergency Department and the surgical ward.

Blunt trauma to the abdomen is far more common than penetrating trauma in the United Kingdom. The mechanisms involved may be related to rapid increases in intra-abdominal pressure from a direct blow or a restraint, such as a seat-belt, direct compression of organs, or shearing injuries induced by rapid deceleration or acceleration forces.

Knowledge of the type and extent of the damage to the road-vehicle, the character of the impact, the use and variety of seat-belts involved, and the presence or absence of intrusion into the passenger compartment, can assist in predicting likely injury-patterns. Eyewitness accounts and reports from Emergency Service personnel can help greatly in providing this information. On occasion, we have found the use of Polaroid photographs of vehicle wreckage or accident scenes to be of help.

For penetrating wounds, the extent and severity of injury is related to the nature and velocity of the weapon. It cannot be overemphasized that the magnitude of external wounding bears absolutely no relationship to the severity of the intra-abdominal injury produced. Stab-wounds from knives, glass, or other implements result in local injury to tissues. Only if associated with major blood-vessel damage are these injuries rapidly life-threatening. By contrast, the injuries produced by high-muzzle-velocity guns or missiles are usually extensive. This is because of the associated effects of cavitation, fragmentation, and internal ricocheting, which can massively compound any locally produced injury.

The nature of the weapons used, the number of shots fired, and the distance between the gun and the patient should be determined if possible, in an attempt to predict the severity of possible injury.

It should be recalled that, during full expiration, the diaphragm can rise up to the fourth intercostal space (the level of the nipples). As a consequence, 'thoracic injuries' occurring below this level may involve the intra-abdominal contents, and vice versa. The presence of alcohol or drug intoxication in the patient, and pre-existing medical problems, should be recognized, together with their likely effects on the patient's perception of, and response to, injury.

Clinical examination

- **Unreliability of clinical examination   Seat-belt sign   Gastric distension   Urethral catherization**

Physical examination of the injured abdomen is less informative and potentially more misleading than for any other body-system involved in major trauma. Even in fully conscious and co-operative patients physical examination alone will fail to detect up to 25 per cent of significant intra-abdominal injuries; while for patients with altered consciousness, whatever the reason for it, this figure may rise to 50 per cent.

All the patient's clothing, including underclothes, should be removed. Take care not to cut through areas involved in penetrating injuries, such as stab-wounds or bullet-holes, as potentially vital forensic evidence may be destroyed.

A rapid, but thorough, examination should be performed, looking particularly for penetrating wounds (both entry and exit sites), abrasions, bruising, and imprinting from clothing. The patient must be log-rolled to ensure that the back, buttocks, perineum, and posterior chest can be fully examined. A rectal examination must always be performed.

Although abdominal pain and local tenderness with guarding are the most reliable features of intra-abdominal injury, their exhibition may be modified in patients with altered consciousness. It is possible for major intraperitoneal damage to occur which yields no detectable signs on clinical examination. Abdominal and/or thoracic injury should be suspected in patients who are more 'shocked' than one would expect from any injuries already detected.

The 'seat-belt sign'—patterned bruising over the abdomen, corresponding to the position of the seat-belt, in vehicle occupants—is often missed or misinterpreted. When present, the frequence of intra-abdominal injury is dramatically increased, even though clinical examination may be unremarkable.

Visceral pain is often poorly localized; but rebound tenderness or guarding are strongly suggestive of significant injury. Such findings should not be attributed to local abdominal-wall injury without further evaluation of the intraperitoneal cavity.

The presence or absence of bowel-sounds is of no value in the diagnosis of intraperitoneal injury. The detection of bowel-sounds in the chest may suggest a diaphragmatic rupture; but otherwise auscultation plays no useful role in the early assessment of abdominal injury. Abdominal girth measurement is entirely useless as an indicator of intraperitoneal bleeding, and is not advised.

Rectal examination is mandatory. The examining doctor should look for blood (indicating bowel perforation or tearing) and the presence of subcutaneous emphysema; should evaluate rectal sphincter tone (to assess spinal injury); and should determine the position and nature of the prostate (to assess urethral disruption).

Gastric distension is present in up to 30 per cent of trauma cases, and is often missed. It may be due to, or aggravated by, positive-pressure ventilation during resuscitation; but it commonly occurs as a result of air-swallowing. Gastric distension compromises adequate ventilation by splinting the diaphragm, and increases the risks of vomiting and pulmonary aspiration. Acute gastric haemorrhage and perforation have also been reported.

For these reasons all severely injured patients should have a nasogastric tube passed and have their gastric contents aspirated. The presence of blood in the stomach contents will also be detected. Patients with facial injury, or those in whom suspicion of cribriform plate or a basilar skull-fracture exists, should have an orogastric rather than a nasogastric tube inserted, to avoid inadvertent intracranial placement.

A urinary catheter should be inserted unless there is a contraindication—for example, blood at the urethral meatus, scrotal haematoma, or the presence of a boggy or high-riding prostate on rectal examination. Catheterization permits the detection of haematuria, and also monitoring of urine output as an index of renal perfusion.

Diagnostic aids

- **Blood tests Radiology Ultrasound/CT scanning Diagnostic Peritoneal Lavage**

Blood tests

Blood tests are of little value in the assessment of abdominal injury. A low hematocrit or a raised white count may be due to intraperitoneal blood-loss or organ-injury, but are of little diagnostic or prognostic value.

A raised plasma-amylase level may result from pancreatic injury, but can also occur after injury to the bowel or liver, or following the use of alcohol or opioid drugs. Conversely, significant pancreatic injury can occur without any elevation of the plasma-amylase level.

Radiology

Plain abdominal radiographs have limited application in the assessment of the patient with an injured abdomen. If emergency laparotomy is needed, radiological studies are only indicated if the patient is stable, and a positive or negative finding will alter definitive treatment.

The commonest radiological investigations required are an erect chest X-ray, a supine plain abdominal film, and a view of the pelvis.

Free intraperitoneal gas seen under the diaphragm on the erect chest film indicates perforation or penetration of a hollow viscus. If it is not possible to sit the patient up, then a left lateral decubitus film may show free intraperitoneal gas, and in this position confusion with the gastric bubble or splenic flexure of the colon is avoided. These X-rays should be performed before peritoneal lavage, as that technique itself causes a small pneumoperitoneum.

Blood within the peritoneal cavity does not have any specific appearances on plain X-ray, although occasionally a generalized ground-glass appearance may be seen.

Retroperitoneal haemorrhage may obscure the psoas shadows, and may also be suspected by associated fractures of the transverse processes of the lumbar vertebrae. Radio-opaque foreign bodies following penetrating injury are usually easily seen.

Ultrasound/CT scanning

Ultrasonography has an increasing role in the non-invasive assessment of blunt abdominal injury. The accuracy of the technique depends principally upon the expertise of the operator. Ultrasound scans are poor at detecting injury to solid organs (such as the liver or spleen), or in defining the sites of hollow viscus trauma. In experienced hands, however, even small amounts of free intraperitoneal fluid can be detected. Visualization of the hepato-renal pouch and the pelvic regions are particularly important, as free fluid is most readily demonstrated at these sites in the supine patient.

Computerized tomography can achieve a diagnostic accuracy of greater than 98 per cent in patients with blunt injury. Splenic, hepatic, and renal injuries, such as lacerations, subcapsular collections, and haematomata, are easily visualized. Free fluid from intraperitoneal haemorrhage or extravasations from the urinary tract are also well seen. Using present techniques, hollow viscus injury is not reliably detected; and duodenal rupture and early pancreatic injuries are often missed.

The accuracy of CT scanning is also operator-dependent, although less so than ultrasonography, while as yet few centres have immediate twenty-four-hour availability of such scanners. At present in the UK the role of ultrasound or CT scanning should be limited to:

(1) patients with blunt abdominal injury who are haemodynamically stable, and in whom there is no other indication for laparotomy;
(2) stable patients in whom peritoneal lavage is contraindicated or has given an equivocal result; and
(3) the further assessment of patients with pelvic fractures, or with urogenital, diaphragmatic, or retroperitoneal injuries.

Diagnostic peritoneal lavage

Peritoneal lavage is the most important adjunct to the assessment of the injured abdomen. The procedure is described on page 161. A direct visual (open) approach is essential to reduce the incidence of local complications and false negative or false positive results. The technique should be performed in the Resuscitation Room in the following categories of patient:

(1) patients in whom blunt or penetrating injury to the abdomen is suspected, and in whom clinical examination is difficult or impossible because of altered consciousness—for example, as a consequence of head-injury or previous alcohol/drug intake;
(2) multiple-trauma patients requiring general anaesthesia for other injuries, or those who have already been intubated and sedated/paralysed; and
(3) trauma patients with unexplained hypotension, or those with equivocal findings on clinical examination of the abdomen, lower chest, or pelvis.

Late pregnancy, gross obesity, and previous abdominal surgery are relative contraindications to peritoneal lavage.

Peritoneal lavage should not be performed in the following groups, in whom laparotomy is essential and lavage would waste valuable time.

(1) shocked patients in whom intra-abdominal injury is obvious or strongly suspected, or those patients who cannot be 'stabilized';
(2) patients with evidence of pneumoperitoneum or diaphragmatic rupture on X-ray;
(3) patients with obvious signs of peritoneal irritation; and
(4) patients with fresh blood or subcutaneous emphysema on rectal examination, or those with persistent fresh-blood aspirates from the nasogastric tube.

Peritoneal lavage should be considered positive (and the patient requires emergency laparotomy) if:

(1) Frank blood or obvious bowel-contents are aspirated from the catheter.
(2) Lavage fluid is seen to exit from a chest drain (indicating

diaphragmatic rupture) or the urinary catheter (indicating an intraperitoneal bladder-tear or bladder-perforation).
(3) The effluent fluid contains >100 000 red cells per mm³.

A red-cell count between 20 000 and 100 000 per mm³ is equivocal. In such cases close clinical review, further investigation by CT or ultrasound, or repeat of the lavage in 2–4 hours (the original catheter can be shut off and left *in situ*) can be considered for stable patients.

Complications associated with peritoneal lavage are infrequent, and all (especially the problems of bowel, bladder, or vessel perforation) are reduced when the open technique is used. False positive results (which occur in 2–3 per cent of cases) are usually related to inadequate haemostasis, which similarly can be avoided by the open technique. Occasionally pelvic fractures can produce a positive result in the absence of intraperitoneal injury.

False negative results (approximately 2 per cent of cases) are usually related to an isolated injury occurring to a hollow viscus—for example, bladder or bowel (especially duodenum)—but may also occur in pancreatic or retroperitoneal injuries.

In the resuscitation of a multiply injured patient, the recognition that emergency laparotomy is required is more important than detailed investigation as to the organ(s) involved. Accurate preoperative diagnosis of the intra-abdominal injury is rarely possible, and is of limited value. The priority must be to have an experienced senior surgical and anaesthetic team involved at an early stage, and to recognize that 'stabilization' of such cases necessitates laparotomy.

Specific injuries

- **Open abdominal wounds   Penetrating objects in situ
  Urethral and urinary tract trauma   Diaphragmatic rupture**

Open abdominal wounds

These wounds are often visually impressive, but are rarely immediately life-threatening. They are commonly the result of slashing injuries from knives, with prolapse of the intestines and/or omentum through the wound. However tempting it may be, do not attempt to push the organs back into the abdominal cavity. The area should be covered with sterile packs soaked in warm saline. If these are not available in an emergency situation then a clean plastic sheet or clingfilm can be used. The object is to prevent drying out and subsequent necrosis of the bowel and omentum, and to reduce external contamination as far as possible. Following further assessment and treatment of other injuries, laparotomy will then be required.

Penetrating objects *in situ*

Most commonly these are knives, fence-posts, or stakes; but any sharp or blunt implement can penetrate and remain embedded in the abdomen if propelled by sufficient force. The object itself may be tamponading or occluding major vessels, and if withdrawn in the Emergency Department uncontrollable haemorrhage may result. Accordingly, as a general rule impaling objects should be left undisturbed, and removed only in theatre during formal laparotomy and exploration.

Urethral and urinary tract trauma

Urethral injuries occur far more frequently in male than in female patients, because of the greater length of the male urethra. The cardinal sign of urethral injury is the presence of blood at the urethral meatus. If this is present, an anterior retrograde urethrogram must be performed before any attempt is made at urethral catheterization.

If there is no blood at the urethral meatus, and the prostate is normal on rectal examination, an attempt to pass a well-lubricated Foley catheter into the urethra can be made. If *any* difficulty is encountered, the procedure must stop, the catheter is withdrawn, and an anterior retrograde urethrogram is performed.

If urethral injury is present and the bladder is distended then drainage by percutaneous suprapubic cystostomy is required. In patients undergoing laparotomy this can be performed at that time.

Injuries to the anterior urethra are commonly caused by direct blows to the perineum, for example during a straddle fall. If the normal fascial planes have been disrupted, urine may extravasate into the scrotum, and extend anteriorly up the abdominal wall.

Injuries to the posterior urethra are most commonly related to pelvic fractures. Up to 20 per cent of pelvic fractures may be associated with a posterior urethral injury. This complication may be clinically suspected by detecting a 'boggy' sensation or a high-riding prostate on rectal examination. Blood may be present at the urethral meatus, and conscious co-operative patients will often be unable to pass urine spontaneously.

In female patients urethral injuries are uncommon, but can occur in association with other perineal or pelvic injury. Vaginal bleeding or laceration should raise the suspicion of urethral injury associated with bony fragments. Because of the short nature of the female urethra, anterior retrograde urethrography is difficult, and more commonly a cystogram with films performed during micturition is required.

Frankly bloodstained urine obtained from a urethral or suprapubic catheter indicates a significant urinary-tract injury. If the patient's condition is stable, further radiographic examination of the urinary tract is indicated. Bladder rupture may be detected by performing a cystogram via the urethral catheter. Up to 250 ml of contrast medium is allowed to flow into the bladder under gravity, and antero-posterior and post-drainage views are taken.

Most commonly vesical rupture results from blunt trauma in patients with a distended bladder (usually due to alcohol intake), and is intraperitoneal. Extraperitoneal rupture more often occurs in association with pelvic fractures (up to 15 per cent of patients with fractured pelvis). Extravasation then occurs into the perivesical spaces. Patients with frank haematuria and a normal cystogram should undergo high-dose intravenous urography. Films taken at 1, 5, and 10 minutes will show whether both kidneys are functioning normally, and delineate renal or ureteric injury. Failure to achieve a nephrogram unilaterally may indicate major vascular or parenchymal damage—or congenital absence of that kidney. The decision as to further investigation in such cases will depend upon the haemodynamic state of the patient and the availability of sophisticated procedures such as angiography and CT scanning.

Patients with microscopic haematuria have a very low incidence of significant urinary-tract trauma, and this finding alone is not an indication for performing an emergency intravenous urethrogram in the Resuscitation Room.

Diaphragmatic rupture

Approximately 5 per cent of patients sustaining blunt trauma to the chest or abdomen have associated diaphragmatic injury. This injury is important because of the frequency of associated injury to abdominal and chest contents, and because of the late complications, which can result in high mortality and morbidity if the injury is missed. The frequency of late complications from missed diaphragmatic injuries reflects the fact that diaphragmatic tears do not heal spontaneously, because the negative intrathoracic pressure during normal ventilation prevents the tear closing. Subsequently herniation of the stomach, bowel, spleen, or liver may occur, with a resulting clinical picture of strangulation or obstruction. Seventy-five per cent of diaphragmatic ruptures caused by blunt injury occur to the left hemidiaphragm, possibly because the right side is 'protected' by the liver.

The 'classical' clinical features of reduced chest-expansion and air-entry, together with bowel sounds in the hemithorax, are rare. More often the presence of associated injuries (especially altered consciousness from head-injury) masks the clinical features of diaphragmatic rupture.

An erect chest X-ray is the most useful investigation, but is often misinterpreted. The most common features seen on the erect chest X-ray include an elevated hemidiaphragm, stomach or bowel loops visible in the chest, and the presence of the nasogastric tube above the diaphragm. Non-specific features, such as haemothorax, shift of the mediastinum, and lower rib-fractures, may be present. On occasion the presence of a herniated viscus in the chest may mimic a tension pneumothorax, and if a chest drain is inserted injudiciously catastrophic results follow. Contrast-medium can be used to outline the position of the stomach and small bowel in uncertain cases. Occasionally, peritoneal lavage may signal the defect when lavage fluid returns from a chest drain; but false negative results are common, particularly with right-sided tears, where the liver may seal the defect.

In contrast to blunt injury, with penetrating injury any part of the diaphragm may be affected. However, because most assailants are right-handed, stabbing injuries are twice as common to the left hemidiaphragm as to the right.

The associated thoracic or abdominal injuries which commonly coexist in patients with diaphragmatic trauma dictate the early operative management. Not infrequently, diaphragmatic injury is found at laparotomy, during careful palpation of the diaphragm in patients with other injuries such as splenic or hepatic rupture.

The pregnant patient

- **Problems with clinical assessment   Priorities   Techniques Risks to fetus   Rhesus negative mothers**

The physiological and anatomical changes occurring during pregnancy can make clinical assessment of pregnant injured patients extremely difficult. In particular, because maternal blood-volume increases by up to 50 per cent, blood-loss may occur before the classical clinical features of hypvolaemic shock are detectable. This relative hypervolaemia may result in some maternal protection; but losses of even 10–20 per cent of maternal blood-volume will critically reduce uterine perfusion. As a consequence, fetal anoxia and distress result, these features being most commonly detected by the presence of a fetal bradycardia (less than 100/min).

Peritoneal lavage can be performed in pregnancy, but must be performed using an open technique, and preferably through a supra-umbilical incision.

The priorities of treatment of intraperitoneal trauma in such cases are similar to those of the standard management of abdominal injury; but it must be borne in mind that both maternal and fetal responses to volume-infusion should be used as indicators of the degree of hypovolaemia and the response to treatment. In the third trimester, if the mother is placed supine, the uterus may compress the inferior vena cava, resulting in reduced venous return to the heart and reduced cardiac output, and aggravating any hypotension. Provided no contraindication, such as an unstable lumbar spine-fracture, is present, the mother should be placed on the left side during the initial resuscitation. Alternatively, if the mother has to remain supine, the uterus may be displaced manually to the left. This may be facilitated by placing pillows under the right side of the trunk and flexing the right hip.

Placental abruption and uterine rupture are uncommon following blunt injury; but both may present with vaginal bleeding and lower abdominal pain, tenderness, and the features of hypovolaemia. Associated fetal distress, with bradycardia, or absent fetal pulses and movements, may be present, depending on the degree of fetal anoxia.

The position of the pregnant uterus dictates the frequency of uterine and fetal injury following blunt or penetrating trauma. Maternal pelvic fractures occurring in the third trimester most commonly result in fetal skull-fractures as the fetal head is engaged; but the gravest risks to the fetus are associated with maternal hypvolaemia or local injury to the uterus or placenta. The risk of uterine involvement following penetrating injury correlates closely with the gestational age of the fetus, and hence with uterine size. In the third trimester direct uterine injury is common, with an associated fetal mortality of over 75 per cent. Clinical features of intraperitoneal bleeding, such as local tenderness, guarding, or rebound, are less commonly seen in pregnant patients.

Injuries occurring in the third trimester with associated fetal distress are an indication for urgent Caesarean section. Similarly, in the event of maternal death the fetus should be delivered by emergency Caesarean section in the Resuscitation Room. The chances of fetal survival are directly dependent upon the extent of the delay between the failure of maternal circulation and delivery. Fetal survival is extremely unlikely if this time-interval is greater than twenty minutes; but the process is justified if any fetal heart-sounds have been detected before the mother's death.

Fetomaternal haemorrhage is important to consider in any pregnant patient following trauma. Kleihauer–Betke analysis (a procedure in which a peripheral blood-film from the mother is stained and examined for fetal red cells) is essential if the mother is Rh-negative. Assessment of fetal well-being by heart-rate monitoring and ultrasonography is not sufficiently sensitive to detect the condition. For Rh-negative mothers in whom documented fetomaternal haemorrhage has occurred, an appropriate dose of Rh-immune globulin should be given, and specialist obstetric advice should be sought.

Further reading

Blaisdell, F. W. and Trunkey, D. D. (ed.) (1982). *Abdominal trauma.* Thieme-Stratton, New York.

Cass, A. C. (1984). Urethral injury in the multiply-injured patient. *Journal of Trauma,* **24,** 901–6.

Chambers, J. A. and Pilbrow, W. J. (1988). Ultrasound in abdominal trauma: an alternative to peritoneal lavage. *Archives of Emergency Medicine,* **5,** 26–33.

Cogbill, T. H., Bintz, M., Johnson, J. A., and Strutt, P. J. (1987). Acute gastric dilation after trauma. *Journal of Trauma,* **27,** 1113–6.

Crosby, W. M. (1983). Traumatic injuries during pregnancy. *Clinical Obstetrics and Gynaecology,* **26,** 902.

Fabrian, T. C., Mangiante, E. C., White, T. J., *et al.* (1986). A prospective study of 91 patients undergoing both computed tomography and peritoneal lavage following blunt abdominal trauma. *Journal of Trauma,* **26,** 602–8.

Fischer, R. P., Beverlin, B. C., Engrar, L. H., Benjamin, C. I., and Perry, J. F. (1978). Diagnostic peritoneal lavage: fourteen years and 2586 patients later. *American Journal of Surgery,* **136,** 701–4.

Fortune, J. B., Brahme, J., Mulligan, M., and Wachtel, T. L. (1985). Emergency IVP in the trauma patient. *Archives of Surgery,* **120,** 1056.

Macfarlane, R. and Pollard, S. (1987). Traumatic rupture of the diaphragm. *British Journal of Hospital Medicine,* **May 1907,** 418–20.

Marx, J. A. (1988). Abdominal trauma. In *Emergency medicine vol. 1* (second edition) ed. P. Rosen, pp. 519–50, C. V. Mosby Co, St. Louis.

Marx, J. A., Moore, E. E., Jorden, R. C., and Eule, J. (1985). Limitations of CT in the evolution of acute abdominal trauma: a prospective comparison with diagnostic peritoneal lavage. *Journal of Trauma,* **25,** 933–7.

Rodriguez, A., Du Prest, R. W., and Shatrey, C. H. (1982). Recognition of intraabdominal injury in blunt trauma victims. *American Surgery,* **48,** 456.

Rose, P. G., Strohm, P. L., and Zuspan, F. P. (1985). Fetomaternal haemorrhage following trauma. *American Journal of Obstetrics and Gynaecology,* **153,** 844–7.

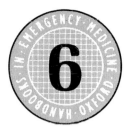

CHAPTER 6

Spinal and skeletal injury

Key points in spinal and skeletal injury

1 Suspect injury to the cervical spine in any patient complaining of neck pain or motor or sensory disturbance, and all patients with altered consciousness or head-injury.

2 Radiographic assessment of the cervical spine must include C1–T1.

3 Pelvic fractures are a common cause of occult blood-loss and hypovolaemia.

4 Haemorrhage from pelvic fractures is often catastrophic and underestimated.

5 The reduction of dislocations associated with evidence of vascular or skin compromise should be performed promptly, and may require to be performed prior to radiographic confirmation if this would involve delay.

6 Splintage of long-bone fractures is essential to reduce pain and associated blood-loss.

Injury to the spine

- Vulnerable sites   Clinical features   Neurological examination
  Prevention of hypothermia   Radiological assessment   Clinical
  management

Injuries to the spinal column occur most commonly where movement is greatest. The cervico-thoracic and thoraco-lumbar junctions are particularly common sites of injury. Although spinal injuries can occur in isolation, they are very often associated with other serious injuries.

Cervical spine injuries are often associated with injuries to the head, and most commonly occur following road-traffic accidents or falls from a height. Important features of cervical spine injury are outlined in Box 6.1, and should be particularly sought in these situations, and in any patient with an altered conscious state:

Box 6.1 Clinical features of cervical spine injury

- Neck pain or tenderness
- Spasm of neck muscles
- Weakness or paralysis of trunk or limb muscles
- Altered sensation over trunk or limbs
- Respiratory irregularity
- Priapism (in the male)
- Loss of bladder or bowel control

Box 6.2 Neurological Examination

1. **Muscle power:**
   - use MRC grading (0–5).
   - examine muscle groups shown in diagram.

2. **Sensation:**
   - to pin-prick, light touch, and proprioception.

3. **Reflexes:**
   - tendon reflexes as shown in Fig. 6.1.
   - anal and bulbocavernosus reflexes.

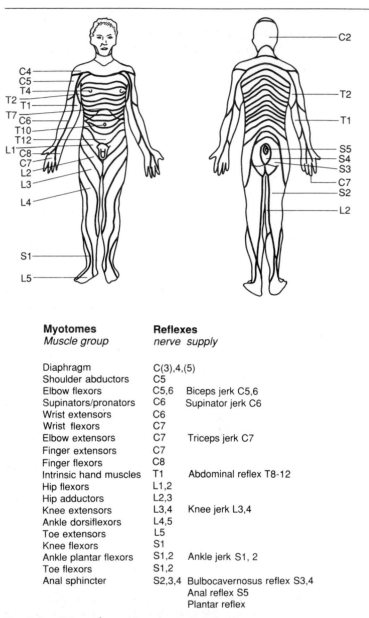

Myotomes	Reflexes
Muscle group	*nerve supply*

Diaphragm	C(3),4,(5)	
Shoulder abductors	C5	
Elbow flexors	C5,6	Biceps jerk C5,6
Supinators/pronators	C6	Supinator jerk C6
Wrist extensors	C6	
Wrist flexors	C7	
Elbow extensors	C7	Triceps jerk C7
Finger extensors	C7	
Finger flexors	C8	
Intrinsic hand muscles	T1	Abdominal reflex T8-12
Hip flexors	L1,2	
Hip adductors	L2,3	
Knee extensors	L3,4	Knee jerk L3,4
Ankle dorsiflexors	L4,5	
Toe extensors	L5	
Knee flexors	S1	
Ankle plantar flexors	S1,2	Ankle jerk S1, 2
Toe flexors	S1,2	
Anal sphincter	S2,3,4	Bulbocavernosus reflex S3,4
		Anal reflex S5
		Plantar reflex

Fig. 6.1 • Dermatomes, Myotomes and Reflex innervation

The level (both myotome and dermatome) and severity of neurological damage must be recorded (see Fig. 6.1).

The deep-tendon reflexes will be markedly reduced or absent in the early phases following cord-injury.

Particular attention should be paid to the perianal area, as preservation of sphincter tone and sensation may be the only signs of an incomplete spinal-cord injury. The anal and bulbocavernosus reflexes should also be tested. The anal reflex is a visible contraction of the anal sphincter in response to a perianal pinprick. The bulbocavernosus reflex is a contraction of the anal sphincter felt by the examining finger during rectal examination when the glans penis is firmly squeezed.

Penile erection (priapism) if present is a rapid pointer to major cord-injury.

Spinal-cord injury is associated with loss of sympathetic tone, which results in peripheral vasodilation without a compensatory tachycardia. Hypotension may develop, and may be associated with a low/low-normal central venous pressure. However, hypotension from other injuries and blood-loss must be excluded and corrected to prevent further ischaemic cord-injury.

A further consequence of the loss of sympathetic tone is that vagal activity to the heart is relatively increased, with symptomatic bradyarrhythmias. This may especially occur during stimulation of the oropharynx by suction. Atropine, in a dosage of 0.6–1.2 mg intravenously, may be required if symptomatic bradyarrhythmias or hypotension occur as a result.

The loss of normal temperature-control, together with peripheral vasodilation, can quickly lead to such patients' becoming hypothermic. This should be anticipated, and the patient should be kept in a warm environment and covered with warm blankets, and if necessary passive rewarming should be commenced.

Radiological assessment

A lateral (cross-table) radiograph of the cervical spine is the most important view. Usually this will require the shoulders to be pulled down to ensure that the C7–T1 junction is included. In some patients a supine 'swimmer's' view will be required to demonstrate this. CT scanning of the neck may be required.

The stability of the spinal-column lesion dictates the risk of associated spinal-cord damage. It must be remembered that

Box 6.3 **Cervical spine radiographs**

Lateral view:

1. Vertebral bodies should be aligned anteriorly, posteriorly, and at the level of the spinous processes.

2. The space between the posterior surface of the anterior arch of C1 and the anterior surface of the odontoid peg should normally be less than 3 mm.

3. The pre-vertebral soft-tissue space at the level of C1–C4 should be less than one-third the width of the corresponding vertebral body. From C5 to C7 the space should be less than or equal to four-fifths the width of the corresponding vertebral body.

4. The odontoid peg should not be deformed or displaced.

Antero-posterior view:

1. The spinous processes should be in the mid-line, and in alignment.

2. The space between each spinous process and the next should be equal.

Open-mouth view:

1. This view allows visualization of the odontoid peg. This should be checked to ensure that it is equidistant from the lateral masses of C1.

2. The lateral margins of the lateral masses of C1 should be in smooth continuity with the lateral margin of the body of C2.

ligamentous injury leading to cervical spine instability can occur *without* fracture. Usually the associated haematoma and soft-tissue swelling will be apparent on the lateral cervical spine film as outlined in Box 6.3, and provide a useful pointer to the lesion.

If the posterior ligament complex and/or neuro-arch is disrupted the injury is potentially unstable. Cervical dislocations are associated with posterior complex injury, and often involve an associated avulsion fracture of the spinous process. This may be seen on the lateral cervical spine radiograph, with widening of the spaces between spinous processes.

Injuries to the anterior longitudinal ligament may follow hyperextension injury and lead to stretching of the spinal cord. Although these injuries may be stable, they are often associated with diffuse cord-damage.

Clinical management

All unstable cervical spine injuries must be secured in skeletal traction. Gardner–Wells calipers are the most suitable for application in the Resuscitation Room. The skin is shaved for 3–4 cm above both ears. Following skin cleansing and infiltration with local anaesthetic—for example 3–4 ml of 2 per cent plain lignocaine, the caliper is applied approximately 2 cm above the ear at the maximal bitemporal diameter. The caliper is screwed through the scalp to grip the outer skull table. Spring-loading of one of the screws should ensure that the correct tension cannot be exceeded. In-line traction is then applied. Between 2 and 5 kg is usually necessary, and the normal cervical curvature can be maintained using a soft neck-roll.

Injuries to the thoraco-lumbar spine produce tenderness over the site of injury in conscious patients. Pain may however be referred to the chest or abdomen because of nerve-root compression and irritation. In patients with altered consciousness a palpable 'gap' as the fingers are run down the back may be the only sign of spinal injury.

Thoracic spine injuries are more commonly associated with complete cord-lesions than those in the cervical or lumbar region. This is because of the limited space between the cord and the surrounding neurocanal in the thoracic region, together with a greater propensity for associated vascular injury at this level. The forces required to produce injury to the thoracic and lumbar regions are considerable: hence the likelihood of associated injury to other structures, especially within the abdomen and pelvis, is high. The clinical recognition of these injuries may in turn be compromised, as symptoms and signs of peritoneal injury may be masked. The importance of additional techniques such as peritoneal lavage and ultrasound scanning is discussed in Chapter 5.

Lateral and antero-posterior radiographs of the thoracic and lumbar spine will be required if any suspicion exists as to injury in these areas. Radiographic appearances of fracture or dislocation in these areas are rarely difficult to interpret, although obtaining good views of the thoracic spine can sometimes be hampered by overlying rib and soft-tissue shadows.

Specific management of these injuries within the Resuscitation Room is limited to ensuring that the patient remains lying in a supine position, and avoiding flexion, extension, or rotation movement during log-rolling or positioning of the patient. Later definitive management of unstable injuries will frequently require internal fixation.

The pelvis

- **General points   Types of pelvic injury   Control of haemorrhage: the MAST suit   Associated injuries to urogenital tract and rectum**

Fractures to the pelvis are second only to fractures of the skull in causing death. The associated haemorrhage is often profound (5 litres is not uncommon), and usually concealed. Sacroiliac joint disruption, usually in a cephalo-caudal direction, damages the medium-sized arteries and veins that accompany nerves in the sacral foramina. These vulnerable vessels lie in the (potential) retroperitoneal space which runs from the diaphragm to mid-thigh. Haemorrhage into this space cannot be adequately tamponaded, and large haematomata may develop. Subsequent rupture of these haematomata into peritoneal space results in massive uncontrolled haemorrhage, which is often fatal. Disseminated intravascular coagulation, due to consumption of clotting factors in the haematoma, is a common accompanying feature. This will add to the already substantial blood-loss. Attempts at open repair of these vessels are often unsuccessful, and haemostatis may require a combined approach, involving use of the MAST suit, application of external fixation devices, and interventional radiological techniques such as embolization.

In the initial hours following major pelvic injury, few external signs may be apparent, and clinical tests such as 'springing' the pelvis are of little discriminant value even in conscious patients. Swelling and bruising in the suprapubic, groin, medial thigh, genital, and sacral areas are late developments, and indicate that profound blood-loss has already occurred.

All patients with major trauma require radiographs of the pelvis, as injuries to this area are a common cause of unidentified haemorrhage. Standard radiographs can usually identify fracture sites; but CT scanning is often required to demonstrate the extent of injury and the accompanying retroperitoneal haematoma. This is of particular importance in the sacroiliac region, where fractures together with displacement can lead to severe haemorrhage.

Types of pelvic injury

Three principal types of major pelvic fracture are encountered:

Type 1: an antero-posterior compression injury, creating a mobile 'butterfly' segment of the pubic rami or disruption of the pubic symphysis. The urogenital tract may be involved in this injury, and the importance of examining the external urethral meatus for blood and of ascertaining the position of the prostate in males is detailed in Chapter 5. Diastasis of 2.5 cm or more at the pubic symphysis indicates disruption, or occasionally complete rupture, of the sacrospinus ligaments, and is invariably associated with major blood-loss.

Type 2: 'Bucket-handle' displacements of the hemipelvis may occur from lateral compression forces—for example, in pedestrians struck by a moving vehicle. Severe disruption to one of the sacroiliac joints and fractures of the superior and inferior pubic rami on one side will be present. Disruption to the pubic symphysis may also damage the urethra and bladder.

Type 3: Vertical shear injuries (Malgaigne's fracture) are associated with the highest mortality from pelvic injury. The nature of the forces applied to complete these injuries mean that associated abdominal injuries and major disruption to vessels around the sacrum are common.

Control of haemorrhage from pelvic fractures: the MAST suit

This device is a three-compartment pneumatic suit which, when inflated, applies compression to the lower abdomen, pelvis, and lower limbs. It was used extensively in the Vietnam War, and in some centres is used routinely for hypovolaemic shock in the pre-hospital setting. Evidence for its efficacy in hypovolaemic shock is controversial; but the MAST suit does have a role in the treatment of patients with major pelvic fractures associated with severe blood-loss. In this situation it provides a direct pneumatic splintage effect, reducing fracture movement. Some degree of tamponade of bleeding vessels also occurs, even at inflation pressures of 30–40 mmHg, that is, *below* systolic arterial pressure.

The MAST suit has two major drawbacks: firstly, it prevents examination of the abdomen. Since these patients are at risk of major intraperitoneal bleeding from visceral injury, where the MAST is to be used diagnostic peritoneal lavage or the decision to perform formal laparotomy will be required before application. Secondly, during deflation and removal of the suit, precipitous falls in blood-pressure can occur. When in place and inflated the suit should only be removed when the patient is in theatre and a surgical team is to hand which is prepared if necessary to perform immediate laparotomy, and occasionally aortic cross-clamping. The deflation process should not be faster than 5 mmHg every minute, and regular checks on the haemodynamic state of the patient must be made, with appropriate adjustments in the rate of volume-infusion.

The MAST suit is at best a 'holding manœuvre', and, not infrequently, haemostasis in patients with major pelvic injuries will require a combination of external fixation-device application and angiography with embolization. If angiography indicates that major arterial bleeding is occurring—for example, from the iliac artery—then open surgical intervention will be required. Haemorrhage from small vessels is more amenable to embolization by means of foam, wire coils, or clots.

Associated injuries to the urogenital tract and rectum

The association between pelvic fractures and injury to the bladder and urethra is well-recognized, and such injuries are fully discussed in Chapter 5. The presence of blood at the external urethral meatus must prompt an anterior retrograde urethrogram prior to diagnostic catheterization. Frank haematuria should be investigated along the lines discussed on p. 89.

Large perineal lacerations may occur in association with pelvic fracture, and require careful early exploration. Rectal examination is mandatory in all patients with major trauma. In female patients with clinical or radiological suspicion of pelvic injury, vaginal examination should also be performed to exclude associated injury.

The severe compressive forces required to disrupt the pelvis can raise intra-abdominal pressure sufficiently to induce injury to the small bowel and rupture of the diaphragm. There is also an association with an increased risk of rupture to the thoracic aorta.

Injuries to the hip joint

• Causes Treatment Complications

The most common hip-injury occurs in road-traffic accidents, when the flexed knee of the driver or passenger has a direct force applied, for instance, from the dashboard, and this is transmitted to the flexed hip. Posterior dislocation of the femoral head from the acetabulum can result. The leg is held in flexion, adduction, and internal rotation. Conscious patients will have severe pain with this injury, particularly on attempted movement, as the dislocated femoral head impinges upon the sciatic nerve. Injury to the femoral vessels and nerve more frequently occurs with anterior dislocations of the hip; but in both cases the risk of avascular necrosis of the femoral head increases with time and with delay in reduction. Associated injuries to the knee and pelvis can make reduction difficult, and usually the procedure will require to be performed with the patient under general anaesthesia.

Femoral fractures

• Complications Treatment Respiratory-distress syndrome
  Associated blood-loss

The femur is the strongest long bone in the body, and it takes

106 • Spinal and skeletal injury

approximately 800 kg of force to produce a fracture of its mid-shaft. Absorption of such force by the body is rarely confined to a single site, and hence femoral fractures are often associated with severe injuries elsewhere. The vascular supply to the femoral shaft is good, and haemorrhage from these injuries can be severe, with over 2 litres of blood lost into the surrounding tissues within the first few hours of injury. For compound fractures blood-loss will be even greater.

The early application of a traction splint, even before radiographs have been performed, is necessary to reduce the pain and associated haemorrhage from the fracture site. There is increasing evidence that an 'aggressive' approach to the orthopaedic management of femoral-shaft fractures reduces the incidence of pulmonary complications, such as fat embolism and the adult respiratory-distress syndrome. The causes of this are multifactorial, including reduction in continued embolism from marrow and reduced needs for narcotic analgesics (and their depressant respiratory effects). In addition, patient mobilization is faster, thus avoiding pulmonary atelectasis and reducing intrapulmonary shunts and the risk of pulmonary thombo-embolic disease.

Box 6.4 Bony injury and associated blood-loss

Chest and abdomen	>2 l
Chest wall	1.0–2 l
Lumbar spine	0.5–2 l
Pelvis	0.5–5 l
Femoral shaft	1.0–2 l
Tibial shaft	0.5–1 l
Shoulder	≥1 l

These values are *very* rough guides only

Injury to the knee, ankle and upper limb

• Dislocation of knee, ankle, shoulder and elbow   Associated risks to vessels and skin   Advisability of early reduction

Dislocation of these joints requires prompt reduction if irreversible damage to surrounding vessels and skin is to be avoided. Around the knee, anterior displacement of the tibia on the femur is the most common displacement, but dislocation in any plane can occur. The popliteal vessels are very vulnerable to injury after dislocation of the knee, and reduction should be achieved as soon as possible in order to reduce the risk of vascular impairment.

Dislocation of the ankle can lead to stretching of the overlying skin, with subsequent necrosis. Manipulation, with in-line traction, under appropriate analgesia will be required, followed by careful splintage. The detection of distal pulses and capillary filling before and after any manipulation is essential, and must be recorded.

The classical appearances of anterior dislocation of the shoulder may not be apparent in the patient with multiple injuries lying supine on the resuscitation trolley. The condition is sometimes initially detected on the routine chest X-ray. Posterior shoulder-dislocation is even more difficult to detect clinically, and may be missed on routine antero-posterior films of the chest or shoulder. It is occasionally the cause of apparent upper-limb weakness, and may follow violent thrashing movements of the upper limb or grand mal fits.

Dislocations of the elbow are usually obvious both clinically and radiologically. In a similar fashion to those around the knee-joint, they are associated with a high incidence of vascular complication. Accordingly, early reduction is indicated, and following the various other life-saving surgical procedures open exploration of the site may be required in patients with evidence of vascular injury.

Compound orthopaedic injuries

- Risks of tetanus, local bony infection and generalized septicaemia Suggested treatments

Any patient with a breach of the skin-surface requires adequate anti-tetanus prophylaxis. The principles of thorough wound-cleaning, debridement, and, where necessary, delayed suture are as appropriate in civilian trauma practice as within the military situation. Anti-tetanus prophylaxis may require the administration of human tetanus immunoglobulin to those patients with at-risk wounds where their imunization status is uncertain.

Broad-spectrum antibiotics are given for compound ortho-paedic injuries to prevent local bony infection or generalized septicaemia. Where dead or devitalized muscle accompanies these injuries the possibility of clostridial infection and the development of gas gangrene must always be borne in mind. In our experience the combination of intravenous benzyl penicillin and a second-generation cephalosporin such as cefuroxime will cover the majority of likely pathogens; but local orthopaedic practice may differ.

Further reading

Bone, L. B., Johnston, K. D., Weigelt, J., and Scheinberg, R. (1989). Early v. delayed stabilisation of femoral fractures. *Journal of Bone and Joint Surgery*, **71**, A336–40.

Grundy, D., Russel, J., and Swain, A. (1986). *ABC of spinal cord injury*. British Medical Journal, London.

Kreis, D. J. and Gómez, G. A. (1989). *Trauma management*. Little, Brown, Boston.

McRae, R. (1989). *Practical fracture management*, 2nd edn. Churchill Livingstone, Edinburgh.

Nallathambi, M. N., Ferreiro, J., Ivatury, R. R., Rohman, M., and Stahl, W. M. (1987). The use of peritoneal lavage and urological studies in major fractures of the pelvis—a reassessment. *Injury*, **18**, 379–83.

Randall, P., Banks, J., and Little, R. A. (1984). Medical (military) anti-shock trousers—a short review. *Archives of Emergency Medicine*, **1**, 39–51.

Ravichandran, G. and Silver, J. R. (1982). Missed injuries of spinal cord. *British Medical Journal*, **284**, 953–6.

Sturm, J. T. and Perry, J. F. (1984). Injuries associated with fractures of the transverse processes of the thoracic and lumbar vertebrae. *Journal of Trauma*, **34**, 597–9.

Yates, D. W. and Redmond, A. D. (1985). *Lecture notes on accident and emergency medicine*. Blackwell Scientific Publications, Oxford.

PART 3

General principles

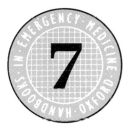

CHAPTER 7

Shock and the metabolic response to trauma

Shock and the metabolic response to trauma: a general introduction

• Definition by cause   Clinical features

'Shock' is a clinical term characterized by impairment of cellular function as a consequence of reduced oxygen availability and utilization.

In the past it was considered that initially oxygen consumption was reduced ('ebb' phase) as part of the normal metabolic response to injury, followed by an increase in oxygen utilization ('flow' phase). More recently it has been shown that the true metabolic response to injury is the maintenance of tissue oxygen-delivery by increased oxygen-extraction.

Oxygen-consumption is directly related to cardiac output and the arterio-venous oxygen-saturation difference. Oxygen-delivery is directly related to cardiac output, and the arterial oxygen-saturation may initially be maintained after injury by compensatory increases in cardiac output. However, if hypoxaemia and hypovolaemia persist, cardiac output and oxygen saturation will fall, leading to a fall in oxygen-delivery. Oxygen-consumption can then only be maintained by increasing the oxygen extraction ratio.

The initial systemic compensatory response to hypoxia is to increase cardiac output, while the pulmonary response comprises hyperventilation and pulmonary vasoconstriction. Reflex pulmonary vasoconstriction in hypoxic regions diverts pulmonary blood-flow to areas of higher alveolar oxygen-concentration. Pulmonary vascular resistance is increased as a result, with additional strain-effects on the heart.

Box 7.1 Clinical features of shock

- Hypotension
- Tachycardia
- Peripheral vasoconstriction
- Hyperventilation
- Sweating

Tissue damage

• Systemic responses   Clinical features   Possibility of further cell-damage

Local tissue responses to injury stimulate systemic responses. In general, the greater the volume of tissue damaged the greater this response. However, the location of injury may also affect the general response, irrespective of the amount of tissue-damage. For example, injuries to the heart and lungs are invariably associated with some degree of hypoxaemia and hypovolaemia because of their special functions, whereas the response to limb injuries is dependent more on the volume of tissue damaged.

The local responses to injury—erythema, swelling, pain, local heat, and loss of function—have been recognized for centuries. These clinical features are directly related to the liberation of mediators, such as endotoxin, histamine, 5HT, bradykinin and the leukotrienes, from injured tissue. These mediators promote vasodilation, increased microvascular permeability, and the clinical features mentioned above. They also activate neutrophils and macrophages, which release further mediators, including elastase, platelet-activation factor, tumour-necrosis factor, and toxic oxygen metabolites. Recent evidence, however, suggests that the true response to injury in man is the maintenance of oxygen consumption, if necessary by increased oxygen extraction when delivery begins to fail.

Hypovolaemia

• Causes   Treatment   Baroreceptor reflex responses Neuroendocrine and metabolic consequences

Hypovolaemia may result from either overt or occult haemorrhage, or as a consequence of generalized increases in capillary permeability as a result of mediator release and prolonged hypoxaemia.

Inotropic and vasodilator agents to increase myocardial contractility and reduce afterload are rarely indicated in the immediate resuscitation phase, and these drugs should not be given unless the ability to monitor their effects is available. Their role is therefore principally in the intensive-care unit and operating theatre, rather than in the Resuscitation Room. Falls in circulating blood-volume lead to a reduction in right-heart filling-pressures. As a consequence, pulmonary blood-flow is decreased, and oxygen-uptake is reduced. Left-heart filling-pressures will also be reduced as a result of decreased pulmonary venous return and cardiac output falls.

The baroreceptors in the aortic arch and carotid sinus will be less stimulated, and their inhibitory influences will be reduced. The baroreceptor reflex responses are mediated via the brain-stem, autonomic preganglionic neurons, and the vagus nerves to the heart, and also by the sympathetic nervous system to the heart and blood-vessels.

A fall in blood-pressure initiates reflex inhibition of vagal activity and an increase in sympathetic activity to the heart. Cardiac output and systemic vascular resistance rise in an attempt to restore the blood-pressure. The cerebral and myocardial blood-vessels do not contract as part of this reflex, and blood is therefore diverted from the periphery to these more important structures.

If haemorrhage or intravascular fluid-loss continues until 20 per cent or more of the circulating volume has been lost, a further reflex is stimulated which can dominate the clinical response. This occurs when stimulation of cardiac C fibres, by distortion of incompletely filled chambers of the heart, produces reflex vagal slowing of the heart and peripheral vasodilation. As a consequence, major circulatory collapse follows. Chemoreceptors in the carotid sinus and aortic arch regions are sensitive to falls in arterial oxygen-concentration. A rise in carbon-dioxide levels or falls in pH increase the sensitivity of these receptors to hypoxaemia. When stimulated the receptors produce tachypnoea, vagal slowing of the heart, and sympathetically mediated vasoconstriction in skeletal muscle. The increase in sympathetic outflow also leads to an increase in catecholamine-release from the adrenal medulla. The neuroendocrine response to shock involves the rapid release of catecholamines, mediated by the sympathetic nervous system, and activation of the renin–angiotensin system. These responses in turn cause release of corticosteroids, aldosterone, antidiuretic hormone, glucagon, insulin, and human growth-hormone. The overall effects of these hormones are to retain salt and water, increase circulating plasma-volume, and maintain blood-pressure.

Adrenalin and noradrenalin increase cardiac contractility, heart-rate, and respiratory rate, and reduce renal blood-flow. The kidney responds by releasing renin from the juxtaglomerular apparatus, activating the renin–angiotensis system and stimulating the production of aldosterone.

Plasma-cortisol levels increase in proportion to the degree of injury until such time as adrenal cortex perfusion falls. The mineralo-corticoid activity of these compounds is relatively small, and certainly insufficient to compensate for all but the most minor circulating-volume loss.

Plasma-glucose rises following injury as a result of increased sympatho-adrenal activity, stimulating the breakdown of glycogen in muscle to lactate. This is released into the circulation pending conversion to glucose in the liver. Glucagon levels are raised, and stimulate hepatic gluconeogenesis and glycogenolysis. Conversely, insulin-secretion is inhibited by the increased levels of circulating catecholamine, and augments the hyperglycaemic response.

In the absence of sufficient oxygen, cells can metabolize glucose to lactate with a release of energy—the process of glycolysis. The reintroduction of oxygen inhibits this process, with the conversion of lactate to pyruvate, which can then enter the Krebs cycle for complete oxidation. Plasma-lactate levels therefore provide an indication of the severity of tissue hypoxia, and of the degree of shock. In the Resuscitation Room these values will not be available, but arterial lactate concentrations have been shown to be inversely related to outcome for individual patients.

Irrespective of the causes of shock, cell-injury and cell-death occur as a consequence of hypoperfusion. With increasing tissue hypoxia, the cell-membrane-bound Na^+/K^+ ATP-ase pump fails. This maintains the normal transmembrane gradients for sodium and potassium, which regulate cell-volume. This change is associated with a fall in intracellular ATP and cyclic AMP levels, and ultimately with cell-death.

In addition, the actions of circulating hormones produced in response to the stress state (catecholamines, corticosteroids, glucagon, etc.) are modified, with further compromise in trans-membrane ionic regulation, and depressed mitochondrial activity. Where prompt resuscitation and re-perfusion occur rapidly, the cellular changes outlined above may be reversed. However, certain organs, such as the brain, kidney, lung, and bowel, are particularly susceptible to hypoperfusion. Further, bowel hypo-perfusion leads to increases in permeability and the absorption of endotoxins, which themselves cause additional cellular injury. The prevention of shock, or, if it is present, its rapid correction, is essential if a vicious cycle of direct cell-damage, leading to the production of further toxic metabolites and further cell-damage, is to be broken. Restoration of circulating blood-volume, oxygena-tion, and ensuring adequate gas-exchange are essential. Attempts to prevent or modulate the effects of shock on various organs are major areas of research interest; but, as yet, appear to be of little clinical value. In particular, the administration of pharmacologi-cal doses of steroids has not been shown to improve mortality or morbidity. Future areas of interest include the use of monoclonal antibodies to a variety of the mediators mentioned.

The time factor

• **Effects of prolonged hypoxia** **Minimization of these effects**

The longer the patient is hypoxic, the greater the tissue-damage that will result. The longer the patient is hypovolaemic, the more tissue is damaged by reduced flow and hypoxia. The longer the patient is in pain the greater the effects of vasoconstriction and tissue hypoxia.

Adequate oxygenation, ventilation, volume-replacement, anal-gesia, and early surgery minimize the hypoxic interval and reduce the overall size of the injury, with consequent reductions in mortality and morbidity.

Further reading

Edwards, J. D., Redmond, A. D., Nightingale, P., and Wilkins, R. G. (1988). Oxygen consumption following trauma: a reappraisal in severely injured patients requiring mechanical ventilation. *British Journal of Surgery*, **75**, 690–2.

Kirkman, E. and Little, R. A. (1988). The pathophysiology of trauma and shock. *Baillières Clinical Anaesthesiology*, **2** (3), 467–82.

Ledingham, I. McA. (1989). Cell therapy in shock: a reasonable prospect or a lost cause? *Resuscitation*, **1989 Suppl.**, 585–99.

Stoner, H. B. (1987). Interpretation of the metabolic effects of trauma and sepsis. *Journal of Clinical Pathology*, **40**, 1108–17.

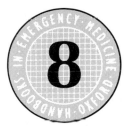

CHAPTER 8

8 Volume-replacement and blood transfusion

Key points in volume-replacement

1 Establish and secure two large-bore IV lines.

2 Take and send blood for Group and Cross-match. Ensure that the blood-tubes and forms are labelled and completed correctly.

3 Prevent further blood-losses by appropriate direct pressure, splintage, etc.

4 Commence rapid infusion with isotonic sodium containing-crystalloid (for example, 0.9 per cent sodium chloride or Hartmann's solution).

5 After 1000 ml of crystalloid has been given, give colloid plasma substitute (for example, Dextran 70 in 0.9 per cent saline, or polygelatin) together with further crystalloid in a ratio of 1:1 while awaiting blood. In life-threatening situations, uncrossmatched O Rh-negative whole blood may be given. Aim to maintain haematocrit at approximately 30 per cent by transfusion of blood, crystalloid, and/or colloid.

6 If experienced in the technique, consider inserting a central venous catheter to measure CVP.

7 Warm all IV fluids (especially blood-products) with in-line warmers. Monitor ECG rhythm, and regularly check plasma-potassium, and if possible ionized calcium.

8 Regularly (at least every 10 min.) measure and record pulse, blood-pressure, CVP, urine-output, and the patient's general condition. The trends in these basic parameters are of greater value in the assessment of volume-replacement than single isolated readings.

9 As blood-loss/-replacement approaches the equivalent of one circulating blood-volume, consider the coagulation competency, and liaise with Transfusion/haematology Services with regard to coagulation screening and replacement.

10 In major blood-loss into the chest or peritoneal cavity. surgical intervention must not be delayed in an attempt to 'stabilize' the patient.

Access to the circulation

- Insertion of initial IV lines   Identification of patient for cross-matching, transfusion and administrative purposes   The significance of delay   Problems of central venous cannulation in multiple trauma

Two large-bore (14–16G, 1.7–2.1 mm OD) intravenous cannulae should be inserted immediately. These should be placed in separate and preferably uninjured limbs. Most commonly they will be inserted percutaneously into the forearm or antecubital fossa veins. North American practice is for one line to be placed above the diaphragm, and one below in the saphenous or femoral vein. This is to avoid any problem associated with mediastinal or cervical injury which may compromise the delivery to the central circulation of intravenous fluid given via the upper limbs. In our experience this is rarely a practical problem; but nevertheless it should be borne in mind in these situations. Depending upon the initial severity of shock and the response to fluid administration, further IV lines may be required.

When the initial IV lines are inserted, 10–20 ml of blood should be withdrawn from one of the cannulae and put into an appropriate blood transfusion cross-matching tube, carefully labelled with the patient's identifying details and the date and time of the sample. If the patient's name and date of birth are not known, he must be given a unique emergency department or hospital number, and this is subsequently used for blood transfusion cross-matching and transfusion and administrative purposes.

Having inserted an appropriate IV line, it must be secured using a piece of 3″ adhesive tape which is put around the arm and can be stuck to itself, not just to the patient's clammy, restless limb. A loop of the IV infusion tubing incorporated in the taping provides a further safeguard against dislodgement. If the cannula has been inserted into an antecubital vein, the elbow must be kept extended by a suitable splint to avoid kinking and consequent reduction of flow.

The importance of rapidly achieving adequate intravenous access cannot be overemphasized. The greater the delay in obtaining intravenous access and volume-replacement, the more difficult subsequent attempts are rendered, as the features of shock develop and peripheral vasoconstriction occurs. Occasionally peripheral percutaneous intravenous access is very difficult or impossible in the arms or legs, and in this situation a venous cutdown or percutaneous cannulation of the external jugular or femoral veins should be considered. The simplest and often most accessible site for venous cutdown is the long saphenous vein at the ankle, where it lies just anterior to the medial malleolus. An alternative site is the cephalic vein as it traverses the anatomical snuffbox in the wrist (see p. 155).

The value of central venous cannulation in multiple trauma is strictly limited. There are three principal reasons why the central venous route is not recommended for volume-replacement during resuscitation. Firstly, the potential complications of pleural puncture resulting in pneumothorax, or subclavian artery puncture leading to haemothorax, are considerable. The complication-rate in patients undergoing central venous cannulation is doubled in inexperienced hands; and there are a variety of possible complications to which the procedure is exposed (Box 8.1). Even in the non-emergency situation experienced clinicians have a 10 per cent overall rate of failed or incorrect catheter placement. Secondly, the flow characteristics of long lines militate against rapid administration of IV fluid. Finally, the reasons for requiring central venous pressure (CVP) monitoring in the early stages of

---

Box 8.1 Common complications of central venous cannulation

- Pneumothorax
- Subclavian artery puncture
- Haemothorax
- Local haematoma formation
- Air embolism
- Hydrothorax
- Hydromediastinum
- Myocardial penetration or perforation
- Local or systemic infection

resuscitation from hypovolaemic shock have to be examined. In fit young adults right-heart filling pressures, as reflected by CVP measurements, correlate reasonably closely with left-heart filling pressures. However, in ventilated patients, or those with acute myocardial or pulmonary injury, this relationship does not necessarily hold. Trends in CVP values may give a more accurate estimate of the adequacy of volume replacement, but a normal or even an elevated CVP does not exclude persisting hypovolaemia.

Overall, in the *immediate* resuscitation of a severely injured patient, measurement of the central venous pressure is unlikely to modify significantly the rate of volume-replacement, or to alter other aspects of patient-care. An important exception to this is in the situation of pericardial tamponade in those patients in whom hypovolaemic shock has been corrected (see p. 72). Accordingly it is important to select those patients in whom central venous cannulation is required, and for it then to be performed by an experienced doctor (see p. 158).

It is well-established that prompt and effective correction of circulating-volume losses will decrease the incidence and severity of complications associated with hypovolaemic shock. In practical terms the three stages of initial plasma-volume restoration, red blood-cell replacement, and the maintenance of competent coagulation can be separately considered.

Initial plasma-volume restoration

- **Choice of fluid   Crystalloid vs. Colloid   Adult Respiratory-Distress Syndrome   The Starling principle**

The choice of fluid for IV administration is a source of much debate. However, it is vital to recognize that the priority is in rapidly restoring circulating plasma-volume, thus optimizing the delivery of adequately oxygenated blood to the tissues. Provided that circulating plasma-volume is maintained, blood-viscosity falls in association with haematocrit. As a result tissue blood-flow and oxygen-delivery can remain normal (or even slightly improved) with haematocrit levels of 30–35 per cent. Only as the hematocrit level falls below 25 per cent does the reduced availability of red cells become an important determining factor in tissue oxygen-delivery. Before blood is available for transfusion the initial steps in volume-replacement involve the administration of crystalloid or colloid fluids.

For the past thirty years there has been controversy as to whether crystalloid or colloid solutions are superior in the management of hypovolaemic shock following trauma. Because of the clinical implications of this debate, some aspects are worth considering in greater detail.

Central to the discussion is the question as to whether the use of these fluids prevents or exacerbates the development of increased intravascular lung water, and contributes to the clinical picture of the Adult Respiratory Distress Syndrome (ARDS).

The principal studies which have been performed relate to comparisons of albumin and isotonic sodium-containing solutions. The simple application of the Starling principle, whereby the maintenance of colloid osmotic pressure by the infusion of albumin or other colloid reduces fluid extravasation into the interstitial space, is inappropriate in the states of shock associated with hypovolaemia or sepsis.

This is because capillary permeability increases dramatically as a result of local trauma and as part of the systemic response to injury or infection. The mechanisms involved include the kallikrein–kinin system, complement activation, and the release of arachidonic acid metabolites and the leukotrienes.

Owing to this increased capillary permeability, albumin and other colloids can escape rapidly from the intravascular circulation into the interstitial space. There is particular concern that escape of albumin across the pulmonary capillary membrane is followed by 'trapping' in the irregular latticework of collagen and elastin fibres which are embedded in the heterogeneous glucopolysaccharide matrix of the interstitial space. This phenomenon may be related to the high negative charge of the albumin molecule and its strong binding capacity. The trapped albumin will then increase the osmotic pressure locally, and lead to interstitial fluid-retention within the lung.

Opponents of these views point out that when crystalloid solutions alone are given for volume-replacement, substantially greater volumes of fluid are needed to restore the patient to the same haemodynamic state than when colloids are used. The argument is then developed by making the point that the infusion of such a large volumes of crystalloid depresses intravascular colloid osmotic pressure to levels where the forces retaining fluid in the circulation are critically reduced.

The few studies which have been performed, albeit in previously fit individuals, indicate that marked falls in intravascular colloid osmotic pressure are not necessarily associated with impaired pulmonary function or increased extravascular lung-water. It appears that this increase in lung-water is prevented by increases in pulmonary lymphatic drainage associated with a reduction in protein levels accompanying the crystalloid fluid replacement.

Elderly patients or those with established shock may be less able to compensate in this fashion, but as yet no adverse clinical effects have been reliably shown.

Outside the lung similar processes occur, with an increase in interstitial fluid, which may result in impaired wound-healing and adverse effects upon gastrointestinal motility and luminal transport functions.

Since colloid fluid resuscitation is volume for volume more efficient than crystalloid solutions it is possible to restore a patient to a normal haemodynamic state more rapidly with them. Overall, however, there appears to be no clinical advantage from the use of albumin as opposed to crystalloid solutions. At present, there are insufficient data concerning the use of artificial colloids as compared to albumin or crystalloids. This means that guidelines as to optimal fluid regimens remain empirical, and factors such as cost and availability are important.

The choice of crystalloid

- 'Normal' saline versus Hartmann's solution   Isotonic versus hypertonic solutions

Firstly, it is important to recognize that dextrose solutions, such as 5 per cent dextrose in water, have *no* role in the management of hypovolaemia. When metabolized, the small dextrose content of such solutions provides little calorific value, while the water content rapidly equilibrates across all the three body compartments, and is therefore inefficient in expanding the depleted intravascular space. The 'free' water aggravates cell-swelling, and this may be of particular relevance in patients with head-injury, in whom cerebral oedema would be worsened.

The crystalloids used most commonly for intravenous volume-replacement are compound sodium lactate (Hartmann's solution) and 0.9 per cent sodium chloride ('normal' saline). Hartmann's solution contains sodium and chloride ions in more physiologi-cally normal concentrations than 0.9 per cent saline, and also contains potassium, calcium, and bicarbonate (as lactate) ions (see Table 8.1). Theoretically the administration of additional lactate ions to patients who already have a lactic acidosis due to hypoperfusion could aggravate this state; but no adverse clinical or biochemical effects have been demonstrated. Thus for practical purposes it seems there is no advantage to be gained from the administration of one rather than the other of these isotonic sodium-containing crystalloid solutions.

Recent reports of the use of hypertonic saline in hypovolaemic shock are of interest. Small volumes (100–400 ml) of hypertonic (up to 7.5 per cent) sodium chloride have rapidly reversed the clinical features of shock, with increases in blood-pressure and tissue-perfusion. The mechanisms involved are complex, and include a vagally mediated pulmonary reflex, producing wide-spread venoconstriction. At present these studies are incomplete and experimental; but if they are confirmed hypertonic saline may play an important role in the early management of fluid-resuscitation in major trauma cases.

Table 8.1 · The constituents of crystalloid solutions used for IV replacement

Concentration mmol/l	0.9% Sodium chloride —'Normal' saline	Compound sodium lactate (Hartmann's solution)	Normal plasma values
Na$^+$	150	131	132–144
Cl$^-$	150	111	95–107
K$^+$	—	5	3.3–4.7
Ca^{2+}	—	2	2.12–2.62
HCO$_3^-$	—	29 (as lactate)	24–30
pH	6.1	6.5	7.35–7.45

The choice of colloid

- Available colloids Anaphylactic reactions Albumin
  solutions Gelatin solutions Dextran solutions
  Hydroxethyl starch

The range of colloids currently available includes gelatins, dextrans, hydroxyethyl starch, and human albumin solution (Table 8.2). Adverse or anaphylactic reactions can follow the administration of any colloid, but the risks appear slight when they are given to shocked patients. The incidence varies according to the colloid concerned, but is of the order of 0.014–0.115 per cent overall, and 0.003–0.038 per cent for severe reactions. Paradoxically, such reactions are more common when they are given to normovolaemic individuals. Anaphylactic reactions are usually associated with histamine-release. The prophylactic administration of H_1 and H_2 blockers has been suggested, although no formal trials have been reported. Our experience is that such prophylaxis is not at present warranted, given the rarity of life-threatening reactions.

Albumin solutions

Albumin is the principal protein in plasma, accounting for 60–80 per cent of the normal colloid osmotic pressure. The commonly available solution has a concentration of 4.5–5.0 per cent, and is iso-oncotic with respect to plasma.

The product is prepared by fractionation of pooled human plasma, sterilized by pasteurization and filtration, and the risks of disease-transmission (such as of human immunodeficiency virus, hepatitis B, and hepatitis non-A non-B) appear to be negligible.

Acute hypotensive reactions have been reported during albumin infusion, and appeared to be due to the presence of prekallikrein activator (PKA) and fragments of Hageman factor, causing bradykinin release. The product is now routinely assayed to ensure low levels of PKA.

Other potential adverse effects of albumin include a negative inotropic effect (due to binding of ionized calcium), reduced urinary sodium and water clearances, and reductions in the levels

Table 8.2 • The composition of commonly used colloid plasma substitutes

	5% Albumin	Dextran 70	Urea-linked gelatin	Modified fluid gelatin	Hydroxyethyl starch
Source	Pooled human plasma	Polymerization of D-glucose by *Leuconostoc mesenteroides*	Bovine bone gelatin	Bovine bone gelatin	Chemically modified maize starch
Average molecular weight (daltons)	69 000	70 000	35 000	35 000	450 000
Colloid osmotic pressure (mmHg)	26–30	66	27	34	19
pH	6.7–7.3	4.5–5.7	7.2–7.3	7.1–7.7	5.5
Half-life	several days	approximately 25 hours	4–6 hours	4–6 hours	days–weeks
Calcium content	—	—	6.25 mmol/l	<0.4 mmol/l	—
Incidence of reactions	1:6600–1:30 000	1:2200–1:84 109 (with dextran/preinjection)	1:700–1:2000	1:325–1:13 000	1:1200–1:16 000
Cost per 500 ml unit	£25–£35	£4–£5	£2–£3	£2–£3	£15–£16

of fibrinogen, prothrombin, and factor VIII, leading to decreased coagulation competency.

Finally, human albumin solutions are markedly more expensive than the synthetic colloids.

Gelatin solutions

The two gelatin preparations currently available are both derived from cattle-bone gelatin by different processes. The resulting gelatin polymers in solution have an average molecular weight of 35 000, and have a colloid osmotic pressure close to that of plasma. The gelatin is suspended in a sodium-containing crystalloid solution. The solutions produce an increase in intravascular volume similar to the volume infused.

The half-life of gelatin in the circulation is 4–5 hours; but this may be modified by hypovolaemia, sepsis, or other situations affecting capillary permeability. The gelatin is finally excreted via the kidneys. Large volumes of gelatin can be given over short periods of time during resuscitation without adverse clinical effects.

Gelatin solutions containing calcium ions can cause precipitation when mixed in the same infusion set as citrated blood, but there is no evidence of haemostatic dysfunction following gelatin infusions, other than dilutional effects. In particular, platelet count and function, prothrombin time, and partial thromboplastin times are unaffected, and there is no interference with blood-typing or cross-matching.

Dextran solutions

High-molecular-weight dextrans are produced by polymerization of D-glucose by the bacterium *Leuconostoc mesenteroides* B512. The molecules are predominantly straight-chain polymers with alpha 1,6 linkages between the glucose units. Two types are commercially available, Dextran 40 and Dextran 70.

Dextran 40 is a 10 per cent saline solution in 0.9 per cent saline, with an average molecular weight of 40 000. The small molecules can enter the renal tubules, markedly increasing urine viscosity and slowing urine-flow. Additionally, reduced glomerular filtration rates and tubular obstruction due to cell-swelling can occur. For these reasons, there is a significant incidence of acute renal failure following infusion in hypovolaemic patients, and Dextran 40 should *not* be used for volume-replacement purposes.

Dextran 70 is a 6 per cent solution in 0.9 per cent saline, with an average molecular weight of 70 000. It has a colloid osmotic pressure of 66 mmHg, and is thus hyperoncotic with respect to plasma. When infused, Dextran 70 will therefore produce a somewhat greater plasma-volume expansion than albumin, gelatin, or crystalloid solutions.

The half-life in the circulation of Dextran 70 is approximately 25 hours, and therefore the volume-expansion effect is more prolonged than that of gelatin.

Adverse and anaphylactic reactions are no more frequent than with other colloids, and their occurrence can be further reduced by the recently introduced technique of hapten prophylaxis.

Dextrans have been shown to interfere with haemostasis, producing reduction in platelet adhesiveness and also in platelet aggregation. This is partly due to a direct effect of Dextran on the platelet endothelium, but is also related to a reduction in the level of von Willebrand factor in plasma. Dextran has also been shown to increase susceptibility of clots to lysis by plasmin.

Finally, blood specimens taken for cross-matching purposes from patients who have been given Dextran 70 may exhibit rouleaux formation. Therefore, wherever possible, cross-matching samples should be taken before any Dextran is administered. If Dextran has been given prior to the sample being taken, the blood-transfusion service must be informed.

Hydroxyethyl starch

Hydroxyethyl starch (HES) is produced from maize amylopectin by a reaction involving ethylene oxide. Different molecular-weight products can be formed according to the degree of acid hydrolysis of the parent substrate, and the number of hydroxyethyl groups can be varied by altering the reaction-time. These aspects are important, in that the rate of degradation of HES in the bloodstream by alpha-amylase is inversely related to the degree of hydroxyethyl group substitution.

The characteristics of HES in respect of volume-replacement are similar to those of Dextran. Its persistence in the circulation can however be extremely prolonged, and some forms have been detected weeks or even months after infusion. The reticuloendoth-elial system is important in the removal and degradation of such macromolecules, and concern exists as to the potential long-term effects of HES on reticuloendothelial and other organ function.

HES solutions do not interfere with blood-typing or cross-matching, but prolonged bleeding times and platelet dysfunction have been described.

Red blood-cell replacement

• **Tolerance of blood loss Composition of blood for transfusion Effects of preparation and storage on red cells**

A previously healthy young adult can tolerate blood-loss of up to 30 per cent of the normal blood volume (approximately 1.5 litres) with relatively few adverse clinical effects, and such deficits can be readily replaced with crystalloid and/or colloid infusion to maintain circulating volume. Acute blood-loss greater than this, or that occurring in previously compromised individuals, will normally require red-cell replacement, and, if persistent, consideration of clotting competency.

The precise composition of the blood supplied will depend upon local Transfusion Service policies and the individual patient. The constituents and nature of commonly available red-cell products used for volume-replacement are listed in Table 8.3. Fresh (less than 24 hours old) whole blood or stored whole blood is becoming increasingly restricted in availability, while specific blood-component therapy is more frequently provided. The indications for using 'fresh' whole blood are debatable; and although some authors strongly favour its use in trauma patients, such opinions are based on emotional appeal rather than objective evidence of efficacy.

Some knowledge of blood-products is desirable, and the indications and problems associated with their use require further examination, since many of the early complications of rapid blood-product transfusion are directly related to their preparation, storage, and administration.

Routinely, 450 ml of blood given by a voluntary donor is mixed with approximately 60 ml of an anticoagulant storage-medium

Table 8.3 · Commonly available blood products

	No. of donations per unit	Approximate volume (ml)	Haematocrit (%)	Shelf-life	Comments
Whole blood (CPDA-1)	1	500	35–45	5 weeks	Provides plasma and non-labile coagulation factors, *but* Factors V and VIII 10–20% normal
Packed red cells	1	300	65	3–5 weeks	0.9% saline may be added to improve flow.
Red cells with SAG-M	1	350	60	5 weeks	Good flow characteristics
Frozen red cells	1	300	70	3+ years	Expensive, may reduce incidence of reactions to white cell antigens
Fresh frozen plasma	1	200	—	1 year	Contains normal levels of *all coagulation factors*
Platelet concentrate	6	200	—	5–6 days	Each 6-pack contains approximately $3 \times 10''$ platelets

containing citrate, phosphate, and adenine (CPDA1). In most centres the white-cell and platelet fractions are then removed, and the red cells are centrifuged to a haematocrit of 95 per cent, the supernatant plasma being removed. Subsequently a solution containing saline, adenine, glucose, and mannitol (SAG-M) may be added, which reduces the haematocrit of the product to approximately 65 per cent and improves transfusion characteristics by reducing viscosity.

Irrespective of the various forms of preparation and storage used, significant changes occur in the red cells. The extent and severity of these changes can be modified according to the exact storage-media and conditions employed.

The important changes include progressive depletion of red-cell ATP and 2,3 diphosphoglycerate (2,3 DPG) levels, leading to structural changes in the cell membrane, with less resistance to deformation and increased fragility. The affinity of haemoglobin for oxygen is increased by a fall in 2,3 DPG, and hence tissue oxygen-delivery is reduced. Potassium leaks out of the red cells, and lactic acid accumulates.

In general these features develop to a greater extent in whole blood rather than in component products, and following transfusion into a recipient they will be at least partially corrected. It is however important to recognize that although a patient's haematocrit and haemoglobin levels may have been restored to 'normal', the function of the red cells in relation to tissue oxygen-delivery may remain compromised for some hours.

Specific problems associated with massive rapid transfusion

- Hypothermia Hyperkalaemia/Hypokalaemia Calcium and citrate changes Blood filtration Other adverse effects of transfusion

Hypothermia

Whenever any intravenous fluid is given at a rate greater than 25 ml per minute, an in-line warming device should be used. This is particularly relevant for blood-products, which are normally stored and delivered at approximately 4° centigrade. Rapid infusion may cause serious cardiovascular complications, including supraventricular and ventricular arrhythmias, together with negative inotropic effects. These effects are further aggravated by the actions that hypothermia has on the hepatic metabolism of citrate, potassium-flux changes induced by the rapid administration of cold blood, and the shift of the oxygen dissociation curve to the left.

Electrically heated water-baths or dryplate blood-warmers can warm blood-products safely to 37°C. In a busy Resuscitation Room, the dryplate devices are simpler to use, less cumbersome, and more reliable.

Hyperkalaemia/Hypokalaemia

During storage, the membrane-bound sodium/potassium ATP-ase pump is inactivated, leading to progressive efflux of potassium from the red cells. The potassium concentration of the storage-medium can rise to 20 mmol/l. Most of this potassium will be promptly transported back into the red cells when they are transfused, provided adequate rewarming occurs. If this does not occur, however, the patient may develop hyperkalaemia, causing cardiac arrhythmias and occasionally cardiac arrest. Although hyperkalaemia may produce classic electrocardiographic changes (prolongation of the PR interval, peaked T waves, and broadening of the QRS complex) these features do not always develop, and they may not readily reflect plasma-potassium shifts.

Later in the management of transfused patients hypokalaemia may also occur, particularly if the administered blood has been stored for long periods. As the red-cell metabolism and the Na/K pump return to normal, the Na/K gradient is re-established across the membrane, with uptake of plasma-potassium leading to hypokalaemia.

Thus it is important not only to monitor the ECG in these patients, but also to perform regular measurements of plasma-potassium.

Calcium and citrate changes

Citrate is one of the components of the anticoagulant storage-medium added to donor blood. Its concentration in the infused product can vary between 2 and 7 mmol per unit given. When

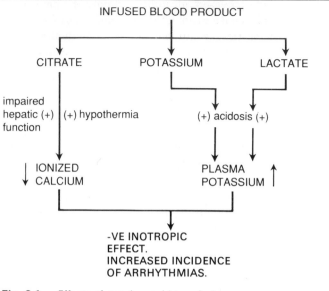

Fig. 8.1 • Effects of massive rapid transfusion

infused, citrate will bind ionized plasma-calcium. Following rapid infusion of stored blood, falls in ionized calcium of up to 40 per cent may occur, and myocardial depression and acute myocardial failure have been reported.

The effects of calcium and potassium ionic shifts are antagonistic in relation to myocardial function. The metabolism of citrate is principally by the liver, and this can be delayed in patients rendered hypothermic by rapid infusion of cold blood-products. Adequate rewarming of such products, together with ECG monitoring and, if possible, measurement of ionized calcium, can detect such changes before clinical problems arise. Provided that adequate blood rewarming occurs, the incidence of such problems will be slight. At present routine administration of calcium 'prophylactically' following the administration of a certain number of units of blood is not advised without such monitoring.

Blood filtration

Leucocyte, platelet, and fibrin debris accumulates in stored blood as micro-aggregates. There is some evidence that ARDS, febrile reactions, complement activation, and adverse effects on reticulo-endothelial function can follow the infusion of microaggregates. However, microaggregates can also be demonstrated in the plasma of trauma patients who have not received any transfusion products, and the relationship between their presence, adverse effects, and transfusion remains unclear.

Micro-aggregates range in size from 10 to 160 microns. Standard blood-filters have a pore size of approximately 170 microns, and therefore allow such micro-aggregates direct access to the circulation. In-line microfilters with a pore size of 10–40 microns are available, but have not been shown to prevent micro-aggregate-induced injury in the lungs or other tissues. From a practical viewpoint, their use slows blood-infusion rate in the resuscitation situation. Specific blood-component products have fewer micro-aggregates than whole blood. For these reasons we do not routinely use microfilters when giving blood-products to multiple-trauma patients.

Other adverse effects of transfusion

Haemolytic reactions related to ABO or Rhesus incompatibility are extremely rare events, and are more commonly due to clerical errors than to laboratory processing. Other haemolytic reactions due to weak antibodies, such as those in the Lewis and Kell systems, are also infrequent in the context of volume-replacement in major trauma, as are those febrile reactions related to white-cell or platelet antigens. Overall, minor allergic reactions have been reported in up to 1 per cent of transfusions, with severe reactions occurring with a frequency of less than 0.005 per cent.

Bacterial and protozoal infection of transfused blood is almost unknown in the United Kingdom, and, following the introduction of specific screening tests for hepatitis B surface-antigen, human immunodeficiency viruses, and syphilis, the transmission of these diseases should not be a major problem.

At present, however, there is no reliable screening test for the agents responsible for non-A, non-B hepatitis. The North American experience is that up to 18 per cent of patients receiving 5 or more units of blood subsequently develop non-A, non-B hepatitis, and of these approximately one-third will go on to develop chronic liver-disease.

Recent research has shown that blood transfusion may alter immune responses in the recipient patient, and increase the incidences of bacterial infection and later tumour-development. These effects are apparently related to the suppression of some components of the reticuloendothelial and humoral defence systems by homologous blood transfusion. Fibronectin and haptoglobin levels have been shown to fall following transfusion, and may have a crucial role in these areas.

While some of the potential problems of blood transfusion would be overcome by autologous transfusion with the patient's own blood, this is rarely practicable in the acute trauma situation. Bacterial contamination of blood within the peritoneal cavity is common, and fat or bone chips may be inadvertently infused after limb-injuries. Furthermore, the equipment and technical support required is considerable.

At present, the benefits of blood transfusion in patients with moderate or major acute blood-loss are overwhelming given the quality and service provided by our Blood Transfusion Services. With the development of newer screening tests for other transmissible agents, and the parallel development of oxygen-carrying blood-substitutes, however, this situation may change over the next ten to twenty years.

Maintenance of competent coagulation

- **Consultation with haematology service Effects of volume-replacement on PT and PTT Thrombocytopenia**

When acute blood-loss and replacement in a trauma patient approaches the equivalent of one blood-volume (approximately 5000 ml), the adequacy of coagulation should be considered. It is vital that there is early consultation with the blood-transfusion/ haematology service. Two particular aspects are worthy of note.

With progressive volume-replacement, the coagulation factors normally present in plasma are diluted. Stored whole blood contains insignificant levels of factors V and VIII, but the remaining factors are usually present in levels exceeding 60 per cent of normal. If component therapy alone is used a progressive fall in the levels of coagulation factors occurs. When between one and two circulating blood-volumes have been replaced elevations in the prothrombin time (PT) and partial thromboplastin time (PTT) will usually be apparent. However, normal coagulation can still occur, despite reduction in the levels of the coagulation factors; and simply correcting the PT and PTT by administering factor concentrates or fresh frozen plasma will not necessarily reverse the bleeding tendency.

In general, fresh frozen plasma has not been shown to be of value either prophylactically to prevent coagulation disturbances, or in bleeding patients, unless the PT and PTT are prolonged to more than 1.5 times the control values. After loss of more than one circulating blood-volume the platelet-count in trauma patients will often fall below the normal limit of $150\ 000 \times 10^9$/l. Spontaneous haemorrhage related to thrombocytopenia rarely occurs with levels above 50 000, and it is the adequate function as well as the number of circulating platelets that is important in maintaining competent coagulation. Platelet-transfusion is usually indicated if the patient is clinically demonstrating a failure of normal coagulation and the platelet-count is less than 100 000. A standard 6-unit platelet-transfusion will normally raise the platelet-count in a recipient patient by 30 000–50 000.

Overall, the magnitude of coagulation disturbance in traumatic hypovolaemic shock is related primarily to the nature of the injury and to the rapidity with which circulating volume is restored, rather than to the volume of blood-loss alone. Replacement of platelets appears to be of greater importance than replacement of coagulation factors. When considering which components are needed the clinical state of the patient should be considered, rather than laboratory measurements alone, and close liaison with the transfusion/haematology services is essential.

Further reading

Collins, J. A. (1987). Recent developments in the area of massive transfusion. *World Journal of Surgery*, **11**, 75–81.

George, C. T. and Morello, P. J. (1986). Immunological effects of blood transfusion upon renal transplantation, tumour operations, and bacterial infections. *American Journal of Surgery*, **152**, 329–30.

Haljamae, H. (1985). Rationale for the use of colloids in the treatment of shock and hypovolaemia. *Acta Anaesthesiologica Scandinavica*, **29**, 48–51.

Hewson, J. R., Neame, P. B., Kumar, N. *et al*. (1985). Coagulopathy related to dilution and hypotension during massive transfusion. *Critical Care Medicine*, **13**, 387–91.

Holcroft, J. W., Vassar, M. J., Turner, J. E., Derlet, R. W., and Kramer, G. C. (1987). 3% NaCl and 7.5% NaCl/dextran in resuscitation of severely injured patients. *Annals of Surgery*, **206**, 279–88.

Isbister, J. P. (1989). Blood component therapy in the critically ill. In *Update in intensive care and emergency medicine 1989*, ed. J. L. Vincent, Berlin. Springer-Verlag, 411–22.

Jones, J. (1987). Abuse of fresh frozen plasma. *British Medical Journal*, **295**, 287.

Kipling, R. and Warner, B. (1987). Replacement of massive blood loss. *Care of the Critically Ill*. **3**, 38–41.

Lancet (1986). Central vein catheterisation [editorial]. *Lancet*, **ii**, 669–70.

Ledingham, I. McA. and Ramsay, G. (1986). Hypovolaemic shock. *British Journal of Anaesthesia*, **58**, 169–89.

Mishler, J. M. (1984). Synthetic plasma volume expanders, their pharmacology, safety and clinical efficacy. *Clinics in Haematology*, **13**, 75–92.

Moss, G. S. and Gould, S. A. (1988). Plasma expanders. *American Journal of Surgery*, **155**, 425–34.

Ramsay, G. (1988). Intravenous volume replacement: indications and choices. *British Medical Journal*, **296**, 1422–3.

Ring, J. and Messmer, K. (1977). Incidence and severity of anaphylactoid reactions to colloid volume substitutes. *Lancet*, **i**, 465–9.

Rudowski, W. J. (1980). Evaluation of modern plasma expanders and blood substitutes. *British Journal of Hospital Medicine*, **23**, 389–97.

Taylor, B. L. and Collins, C. (1988). The management of massive haemorrhage. *British Journal of Hospital Medicine*, **40**, 104–10.

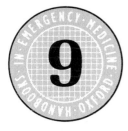

CHAPTER 9

Transfer of the trauma patient

The transfer of the multiply
injured patient 145

Further reading 148

NEATH GENERAL HOSPITAL

Transfer of the multiply injured patient

- Further management and indications for referral and transfer Complications associated with transfer

The resuscitation of multiply injured patients is complete only when all surgery has been accomplished and the patient is haemodynamically stable. If unnecessary deaths and complications are to be avoided, this must be achieved in the shortest possible time.

Box 9.1 Information which will be requested by the receiving centre at the time of telephone consultation

1. Patient's name, age, and previous health status (if available)

2. The pulse, blood-pressure, and respiratory rates (at scene, on arrival, and at present)

3. Glasgow Coma Scale (at scene, on arrival, and at present)

4. External signs of head-injury, lateralizing signs (limb weakness, pupil responses)

5. The assessment and treatment required for other body systems, the amounts of IV fluids given, and the haemodynamic responses obtained

6. The results of radiographic investigation, CT scans, and arterial blood-gas analysis

---

The optimal outcome occurs when a patient is taken directly and swiftly to a centre where all relevant specialties are on site, and further transfer is unnecessary. Few centres in the United Kingdom have these facilities. Most frequently, patients require to be transferred to receive neurosurgical expertise. However, it has been shown the whenever multiply injured patients are transferred, there is an associated significant increase in mortality. This is in part related to inadequate levels of resuscitation achieved prior to and during the transfer. Patients must never be transferred without consultation, no matter how strong the urge to 'cut and run'.

In general, if anything can go wrong in transfer, it will. The patient's airway must be secured, if necessary with endotracheal intubation and positive-pressure ventilation. Pneumothoraces or chest-injuries likely to be associated with a pneumothorax must have tube thoracostomy performed before transfer.

Acute gastric dilatation is a common accompaniment of head and other injuries, and pulmonary aspiration can occur. A nasogastric tube (or orogastric tube if the cribriform plate is thought to have been damaged) should be inserted, and the gastric contents should be aspirated.

Thoracostomy tubes must never be clamped, as a tension pneumothorax can occur rapidly. Underwater-seal drainage bottles are clumsy and prone to tipping and spilling. The use of drainage bags with integral one-way valves is much more practical for inter-hospital transfer. If underwater-seal bottles have to be used they must be kept below the level of the patient, to prevent aspiration of water into the chest.

Ensure that enough oxygen is available for the journey. A standard large 'F' cylinder contains 1360 litres of oxygen. This will last less than 3 hours at a rate of administration of 10 litres per minute. Oxygen-driven portable ventilators will consume up to 21 litres per minute. If 'no airmix' is selected, a full cylinder will only last for approximately 60 minutes.

Intravenous lines must be secured, and adequate amounts of blood and other intravenous fluids must be available. If arterial lines have been placed, they should be flushed with heparinized saline, and sealed during transfer. The dangers associated with accidental disconnection of arterial lines far outweigh any benefits, unless the staff involved in transfer have special experience in their management. The site of entry of arterial or central venous lines must not be obscured, to ensure adequate observation and recognition of leakage or disconnection.

A fully charged portable ECG monitor/defibrillator should be available, and, if available, a portable pulse oximeter may give warning of impending deterioration, particularly when the noise and movement of the vehicle prevent accurate examination. The journey should be smooth and safe, and sudden changes in direction, accelerations, and decelerations should be avoided.

These factors should be stressed to the ambulance crew, together with the nature of the case and the reason for transfer.

In our experience, the use of helicopters for transfers in an urban or semi-urban environment is of little additional benefit. The reduced journey-time is usually more than offset by restrictions in availability and in access to helicopter landing-sites. In addition, monitoring of patients in many helicopters is difficult because of noise and vibration, and there are limits on the number of staff that may accompany the patient.

Completed case-notes, radiographs, blood-results, and cross-matched blood should accompany the patient, together with the transfer-case and its contents, listed in Box 9.2.

Box 9.2 Contents of the adult transfer-case

Airway

Self-expanding bag and mask

Oxygen-mask and tubing

Yankauer and soft tracheal suction catheters

Laryngoscope, together with spare batteries and bulb

Guedel airways, sizes 2, 3, and 4

Cuffed endotracheal tubes, sizes 7.5 to 9.5 inclusive

Endotracheal-tube introducer

Macbic clamp

10 ml syringe

McGill forceps

Bandage/tape for securing endotracheal tube

Minitrach set

Catheter mount

Thoracostomy

Thoracostomy tubes size 28 × 2

Drainage bags × 2

Disposable scalpel and blade, size 10, × 2

2/0 silk suture on curved hand-held needle × 2

Spencer–Wells forceps × 2

Gauze dressing

'Sleek' adhesive tape

Sterile latex gloves

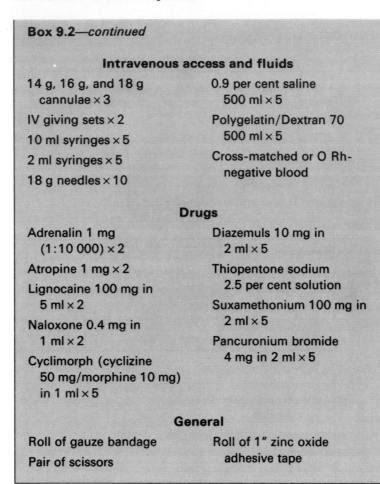

Box 9.2—*continued*

Intravenous access and fluids

14 g, 16 g, and 18 g cannulae × 3	0.9 per cent saline 500 ml × 5
IV giving sets × 2	Polygelatin/Dextran 70 500 ml × 5
10 ml syringes × 5	
2 ml syringes × 5	Cross-matched or O Rh-negative blood
18 g needles × 10	

Drugs

Adrenalin 1 mg (1:10 000) × 2	Diazemuls 10 mg in 2 ml × 5
Atropine 1 mg × 2	Thiopentone sodium 2.5 per cent solution
Lignocaine 100 mg in 5 ml × 2	Suxamethonium 100 mg in 2 ml × 5
Naloxone 0.4 mg in 1 ml × 2	Pancuronium bromide 4 mg in 2 ml × 5
Cyclimorph (cyclizine 50 mg/morphine 10 mg) in 1 ml × 5	

General

Roll of gauze bandage	Roll of 1″ zinc oxide adhesive tape
Pair of scissors	

Further reading

Ehrenwerth, J., Sorbo, S., and Hackel, A. (1986). Transport of critically ill adults. *Critical Care Medicine*, **14**, 543–7.

Gentleman, D. and Jennett, B. (1981). Hazards of interhospital transfer of comatose head injured patients. *Lancet*, **ii**, 853–5.

Waddell, G., Scott, P. D. R., Lees, N. W., and Ledingham, I. McA. (1975). Effects of ambulance transport in critically ill patients. *British Medical Journal*, **1**, 386–9.

Wright, I. H., McDonald, J. C., Rogers, P. N., and Ledingham, I. McA. (1988). Provision of facilities for secondary transport of seriously ill patients in the United Kingdom. *British Medical Journal*, **296**, 543–5.

PART 4

Practical procedures; and a note on Last Things

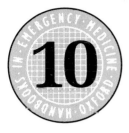

Practical procedures

Practical procedures: general points

The Resuscitation Room is *not* the place for an inexperienced doctor to perform for the first time the various procedures described in this section. Some of these techniques can and should be taught initially on cadavers in the Anatomy and Post-mortem Rooms, or on manikins. Once complete familiarity is achieved, they can then be translated to appropriate patients in elective situations prior to their use in the Resuscitation Room. When these techniques are being performed on conscious patients, appropriate explanation, reassurance, and local anaesthesia must be used.

In the pre-hospital environment and the Resuscitation Room, normally followed sterile precautions may not always be practicable, because of the urgency and nature of the clinical situation. However, when possible the operator should use standard sterile procedure, with hand-washing and the use of gloves, gowns, and drapes, together with appropriate skin-preparation of the patient. With the recognized hazards to emergency staff from agents such as hepatitis B, human immunodeficiency virus, and non-A, non-B hepatitis, the importance of adequate universal staff precautions cannot be overemphasized.

Venous cutdown

Venous cutdown may be required when the insertion of percutaneous cannulae cannot be achieved and venous access is urgently required. The most commonly used sites are the long saphenous vein at the ankle, the median cubital vein in the antecubital fossa, and the saphenofemoral vein at the groin (Figs. 10.1–10.3). Appropriate skin-cleaning and local anaesthesia should be used as necessary.

When the technique is being performed in the antecubital or ankle regions, a proximal tourniquet should be applied to aid venous filling and hence identification.

The saphenous vein lies in a constant position at the ankle, just anterior to the medial malleolus.

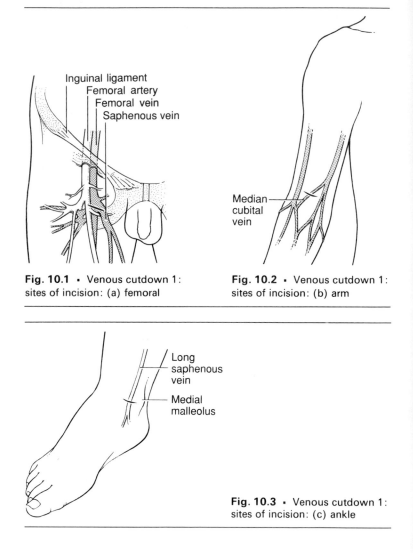

Fig. 10.1 • Venous cutdown 1: sites of incision: (a) femoral

Fig. 10.2 • Venous cutdown 1: sites of incision: (b) arm

Fig. 10.3 • Venous cutdown 1: sites of incision: (c) ankle

A small (2–3 cm) transverse incision is made at the level of the medial malleolus, and the vein is cleared from surrounding tissues using blunt dissection with haemostats (Fig. 10.4). Two loops of 3/0 chromic catgut are passed under the vein, and the distal suture is tied. The proximal suture is held with forceps to stabilize the vein, while a small V-shaped incision is made in the wall of the

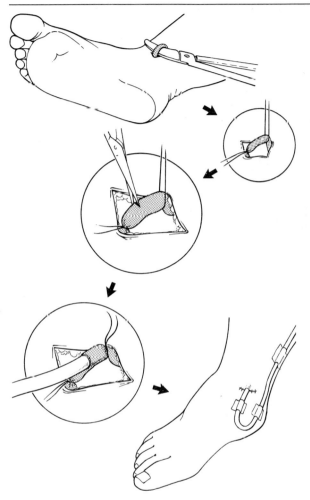

Fig. 10.4 • Venous cutdown 2: procedure sequence

vein with sharp-pointed scissors. The cannula is then inserted, and secured by tying the proximal suture around the vein containing it.

The proximal tourniquet is removed, and infusion of fluid is commenced.

The incision is then closed with 3/0 or 4/0 silk or nylon sutures.

In the emergency situation skin-tunnelling so that the cannula exits at a different site from the initial wound is not appropriate; but the catheter must be secured to the skin in a loop with adhesive tape, so that movement of the drip-tubing will not lead to dislodgement.

When the procedure is performed at the saphenofemoral vein in the groin the incision is made approximately 2 finger-breadths below the inguinal ligament, just medial to the pulsation of the femoral artery. The incision should be approximately 5 cm long.

Using blunt dissection the subcutaneous tissue and fascia are cleared. The saphenofemoral vein lies immediately below Scarpa's fascia. It should be dissected free, and then the above technique should be followed.

In extremis, for patients requiring rapid and massive amounts of volume-replacement, the end of a sterile intravenous giving set can be cut obliquely and used instead of a standard intravenous cannula. This enables infusion rates of up to 1 litre per minute to be achieved by this route.

Central venous cannulation

Central venous cannulation may be indicated following major trauma to assess right-heart filling-pressures and the adequacy of volume-replacement. In exceptional circumstances it may be required for the administration of drugs or fluids where other forms of venous access cannot be achieved.

The technical difficulties involved are considerable, with potentially life-threatening complications (see p. 125). It is important that the operator is entirely familiar with the superficial and deep anatomy concerned, and approaches to the internal jugular or subclavian veins from the neck should never be undertaken by the inexperienced (Fig. 10.5). If necessary a long intravenous cannula can be inserted via the median cubital vein at the elbow, and fed proximally into the superior vena cava via the subclavian vein.

It is recommended that wherever possible the right side of the neck should be used, to avoid possible puncture of the thoracic duct. If an intercostal tube is however already *in situ* (for example,

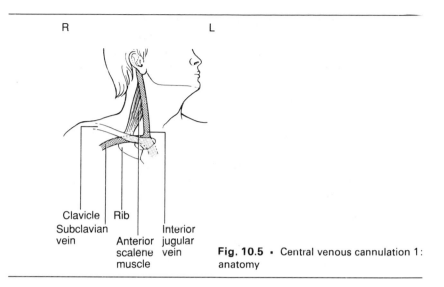

Clavicle | Rib
Subclavian | | Interior
vein | Anterior | jugular
scalene | vein
muscle

Fig. 10.5 • Central venous cannulation 1: anatomy

for the drainage of a pneumo- or haemothorax) then the same side should be considered for cannulation rather than risk a pneumothorax on the other (uninjured) side.

Techniques using a guidewire (the Seldinger procedure) are to be preferred, because the risks of pneumothorax and haemorrhage are reduced.

Internal jugular approach

The internal jugular vein runs in a straight line deep to the sternomastoid muscle, between the mastoid process and the sternal end of the clavicle (Fig. 10.6).

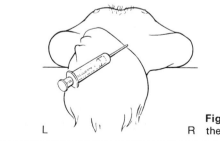

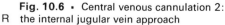

Fig. 10.6 • Central venous cannulation 2: the internal jugular vein approach

The patient should be placed with a 10°–15° head-down tilt. The head is turned away from the site of the venepuncture. When appropriate, local anaesthetic should be used.

The needle is inserted at the mid-point between the sternal head of the clavicle and the mastoid process, at an angle of 30°–40° to the skin, just medial to the sternomastoid muscle and advanced inferiorly and laterally towards the ipsilateral nipple. The vein is normally located at a depth of 2–3 cm, and entry is confirmed by aspirating blood.

The syringe is carefully disconnected, leaving the needle *in situ*, and the flexible tip of the guidewire is passed through the needle so that at least 10 cm of the wire lies within the internal jugular vein.

A small skin incision is made at the site where the wire passes through the skin, and the tapered venous cannula is passed over the wire, through the skin, and into the vein. It is important to check that the free proximal end of the guidewire is always visible and secured.

The guidewire is then withdrawn from the cannula. Confirmation that the cannula lies in the vein is achieved by ensuring that blood can be aspirated from the cannula.

The cannula is then connected to the intravenous infusion set, and must be secured to the skin using an appropriate suture and tape.

Supraclavicular approach to the subclavian vein

The sternal and clavicular heads of the sternomastoid muscle form a triangle whose base is the clavicle.

Where appropriate, local anaesthetic is infiltrated into the skin at the angle between the clavicular head of the sternomastoid and the clavicle.

The needle is inserted at an angle of 45° to the skin and to the clavicle at this site, and advanced towards the manubriosternal joint (Fig. 10.7).

The subclavian vein is normally entered at a depth of 3–4 cm. Subsequently, the process outlined above is followed.

The hazards of pneumothorax and inadvertent arterial puncture leading to haemothorax are the commonest complications for both techniques. Local bleeding from inadvertent puncture of the

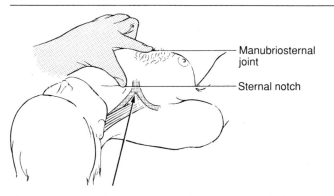

Fig. 10.7 • Central venous cannulation 3: the supraclavicular approach to the subclavian vein

carotid or subclavian arteries can produce rapidly expanding haematomata of the neck, which may on occasion lead to airway obstruction. Direct local pressure should be applied to prevent this occurring. Air embolism is a potential risk, particularly in hypovolaemic patients, but can be minimized by the head-down tilt position. Following successful or unsuccessful attempts at central venous cannulation, a chest X-ray is mandatory, to detect potential complications.

Diagnostic peritoneal lavage

The indications for performing lavage in trauma patients are outlined on p. 86. Prior to the procedure's being performed, a naso- or orogastric tube should be passed and the stomach contents should be aspirated. A urinary catheter should be inserted to ensure that the bladder is empty (Fig. 10.8).

The patient should be placed supine, with a 5°–10° head-down tilt. Following local skin antisepsis, the skin and subcutaneous tissues are infiltrated with 1 per cent lignocaine containing 1/200 000 adrenalin at a site 2–3 cm below the umbilicus in the mid-line. A 3 cm longitudinal mid-line incision is made.

Under direct vision, the subcutaneous tissues are dissected

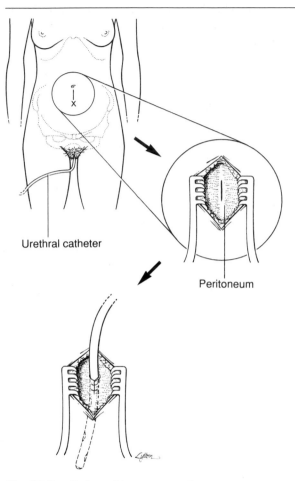

Fig. 10.8 • Peritoneal lavage: procedure sequence

using a blunt technique, the linea alba is incised, and the peritoneum is visualized. Meticulous haemostatis should be assured, to prevent false positive results occurring.

The peritoneum is grasped between two pairs of artery forceps, and a small hole is made using fine scissors or a scalpel.

The peritoneal dialysis catheter (without the stilette) is then inserted into the peritoneal cavity under direct vision and advanced towards the pelvis.

The catheter should then be aspirated gently, using a 20 ml syringe. If blood is obtained on aspiration, the test is positive, and further lavage is unnecessary.

If no blood is aspirated from the catheter, one litre of warmed (approximately 40° centigrade) sterile normal saline is run into the peritoneal cavity through an intravenous infusion set.

The patient should be gently rolled from side to side and tilted from the head-down position to a neutral position to ensure that the lavage fluid has access to all of the intraperitoneal cavity. The fluid is then siphoned from the intraperitoneal cavity under gravity, and if possible 750 ml should be recovered.

An aliquot is sent for laboratory analysis to determine the red-cell count.

In equivocal cases the cannula can be left *in situ* and the lavage can be repeated later provided the patient remains stable. With a negative result, the cannula should be removed and the wound closed, ensuring appropriate suture of the peritoneum, linea alba, and skin.

Chest drainage

If time and the patient's clinical condition permit, an erect chest X-ray should be performed before needle thoracocentesis or intercostal drainage, as conditions such as diaphragmatic rupture, gastric dilation, or bullous emphysema can mimic a pneumothorax.

In a patient who has a life-threatening tension pneumothorax, needle thoracocentesis should be performed prior to the formal insertion of an intercostal chest drain.

A large (12–14 gauge) needle and cannula are inserted into the second intercostal space in the mid-clavicular line on the appropriate side. When the needle is removed, leaving the cannula *in situ*, there is a characteristic hiss of air escaping from the thorax as the 'tension' is relieved. Subsequently tube thoracostomy will be required.

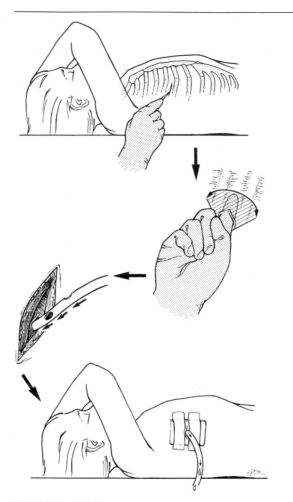

Fig. 10.9 • Chest drainage: procedure sequence

Intercostal chest drain insertion (Tube thoracostomy)

The optimal site of insertion is the fourth intercostal space, just anterior to the mid-axillary line.

The patient should be supine, with the arm fully abducted. Following skin-preparation, the skin and subcutaneous tissue are infiltrated with local anaesthetic down to, and including the parietal pleura.

A 2–3 cm horizontal incision is made parallel to the long axis of the ribs.

The incision must be long enough to allow the insertion of a finger, and is carried down to the intercostal muscles, which are then divided by blunt dissection with scissors and/or scalpel along the superior surface of the fifth rib. The parietal pleura is entered, and confirmation of the location is obtained by inserting a gloved finger into the chest. The finger is swept round to ensure that the lung is not adherent at this site. If adhesions are present, an alternative site, for example, the second intercostal space in the mid-clavicular line, should be used.

The tip of the intercostal drainage tube (26–30 FG) is then grasped with a large haemostat and inserted into the thoracic cavity alongside the finger, which is used to direct it superiorly. The thoracostomy tube is then connected to the underwater-seal drain, and confirmation that the tube is in the thoracic cavity is obtained by observing the level of water in the drainage-bottle to rise and fall with respiration.

The tube is then secured with a suture, and further sutures are placed to close the skin incision.

The wound is dressed, and the tube further secured by adhesive tapes.

It is important to tape the connections of the intercostal drainage cannula to the underwater-seal drain to prevent accidental disconnection.

Following the procedure, a chest X-ray is performed to confirm the site of the tube within the thorax and the resolution of the pneumohaemothorax.

A Heimlich valve may be used instead of an underwater-seal drain in patients with a pneumothorax; but in our experience many trauma patients have an associated haemothorax, and blood can clog up the flutter-mechanism in the valve. In the pre-hospital situation, a urine-drainage bag attached to the thoracostomy tube can provide a temporary drainage-mechanism.

A laterally placed chest drain will drain both air and blood adequately, as when the lung expands any residual pleural space is obliterated. A possible exception to this can occur where a large air-leak is present, for instance from a major bronchial tear, such that the lung on that side does not re-expand.

There is no evidence that any tamponading effect on a haemothorax can be obtained by clamping off an intercostal chest drain. Even on first principles this would not be expected, since the potential volume of the hemithorax exceeds the normal circulating blood-volume.

Chest drains are commonly mismanaged during transportation. All connections must be securely taped. The tubing must *never* be clamped. To ensure that syphoning of the contents does not occur the underwater-seal bottle must not be lifted above the level of the intercostal tube.

Femoral nerve-block

This local anaesthetic technique is extremely useful in patients who have pain associated with femoral fractures. It is a simple technique which can rapidly provide good analgesia in patients who may require manipulation or other movement related to splintage.

Femoral nerve-block should not be performed where fractures of the lower limb are associated with a vascular or neurological problem, or where the patient is known to be hypersensitive to the local anaesthetic agent used.

The pubic tubercle and anterior superior iliac spine are identified on the appropriate side. The femoral artery can be palpated midway between these points, just below the inguinal ligament (Fig. 10.10).

Following skin-preparation, the needle is inserted approximately 1 cm lateral to the femoral artery pulsation. A characteristic loss of resistance may be felt as the needle goes through the fascia lata and fascia iliaca (Fig. 10.11). After aspirating to ensure that inadvertent vessel-puncture has not occurred, the anaesthetic is then injected.

As anaesthetic agents 0.5 per cent bupivacaine or 1 per cent lignocaine with adrenalin can be used. As the anaesthetic is injected, the needle should be fanned laterally, after careful aspiration.

If the needle touches the nerve, the patient may complain of sharp pain or paraesthesia down the leg, in which case the needle should be withdrawn slightly and the local anaesthetic should be injected slowly.

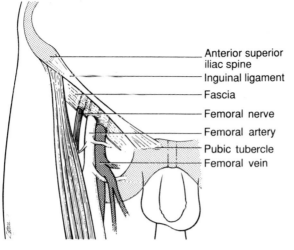

Anterior superior
iliac spine

Inguinal ligament

Fascia

Femoral nerve

Femoral artery

Pubic tubercle

Femoral vein

Fig. 10.10 • Femoral nerve-block 1: anatomy

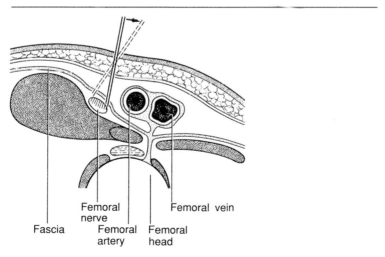

Femoral
nerve

Femoral vein

Fascia   Femoral   Femoral
            artery   head

Fig. 10.11 • Femoral nerve-block 2: site of anaesthesia (cross-section)

Anaesthesia usually develops within five minutes. Manipulation or other movements should be withheld until adequate analgesia has been achieved.

Advanced airway management

The maintenance of a competent upper airway and adequate ventilation is rarely a problem in conscious patients. However, for those with altered consciousness, particularly if this is associated with vomiting or anatomical disturbance of the upper airway, advanced airway techniques are often needed. The attendant risks of increasing intracranial pressure, catecholamine-release, and vagal responses, together with the possibility of causing or exacerbating cervical cord-injury, necessitate that such procedures are performed only by doctors experienced in the technique and in the management of potential complications.

Where the possibility of cervical spine-injury exists and time permits, a lateral cervical spine X-ray is invaluable. While a normal film does not exclude cervical cord-damage, it will indicate whether the cervical spine is sufficiently stable to allow optimal airway-management. In our view, for experienced doctors the risk of orotracheal intubation inducing further cord-injury in apnoeic or near-apnoeic trauma patients is outweighed by the necessity to treat the coexistent hypoxia and hypoventilation. Irrespective of the technique used it is essential to check:

- that adequate, functioning suction-apparatus, Yankauer, and soft-suction catheters are immediately to hand.
- that the laryngoscope is working (especially check batteries and bulb).
- that the patient is preoxygenated, and if necessary ventilated with a bag and mask.
- that the patient is positioned to facilitate visualization of the airway landmarks (see Fig. 10.12, p. 170).
- that a selection of endotracheal tubes, pre-cut to length and having had their balloon cuffs checked to exclude leakage, is available.

Endotracheal intubation

Where possible, oral endotracheal intubation is recommended. The visualization of the larynx and vocal cords is better, a larger-diameter endotracheal tube can be inserted, there is less risk of epistaxis or oropharyngeal haemorrhage, and there is a higher success rate. The presence or possibility of a coexistent cervical spine-fracture is a relative, but not an absolute, contraindication for oral endotracheal intubation. In our experience it is preferable for an assistant to stabilize the head and neck while intubation is performed rather than to fail to achieve an adequate airway. Nasotracheal intubation or cricothyrotomy are possible alternative techniques in this situation.

An assistant should maintain digital pressure on the cricoid cartilage to reduce the risk of vomiting and aspiration (Sellick manœuvre). This procedure also displaces the larynx posteriorly, aiding visualization.

The laryngoscope is held in the left hand, and introduced just to the right of the mid-line. It is important to avoid trauma to the teeth or lips.

The tongue and jaw are lifted upwards as the tip of the laryngoscope is advanced into the vallecula (Figs. 10.12 and 10.13). Gentle traction upwards elevates the epiglottis, to reveal the larynx and vocal cords.

A lubricated endotracheal tube is then passed under direct vision through the vocal cords into the trachea.

Suitable endotracheal tube sizes are: 8.5–9.5 mm for adult males, 7.5–8.5 mm for adult females, and 7.0 mm for small adults or adolescents.

The cuff of the endotracheal tube is then inflated sufficiently to prevent escape of air around the tube during ventilation. The digital pressure to the cricoid cartilage can now be withdrawn, and ventilation can start. Auscultate both sides of the chest to ensure that air-entry is symmetrical.

The endotracheal (E-T) tube should be secured to the patient's face using adhesive tape.

An oropharyngeal (Guedel) airway is inserted, to prevent the patient biting the E-T tube.

A proportion of patients need to be sedated and/or paralysed to permit endotracheal intubation and ventilation. The precise

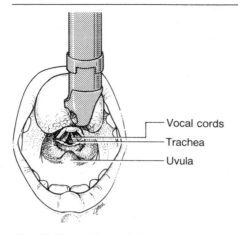

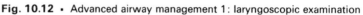

Fig. 10.12 • Advanced airway management 1: laryngoscopic examination

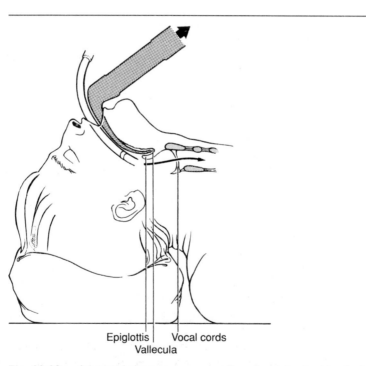

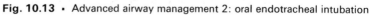

Fig. 10.13 • Advanced airway management 2: oral endotracheal intubation

indications for this vary, but they include those who are agitated because of hypoxia, head-injury, or alcohol/drug intoxication, and those with major thoracic injuries, especially where a 'flail' segment is present.

Such patients should be pre-oxygenated, and appropriate positioning of the head and neck should be ensured. The assistant should apply pressure to the cricoid cartilage. A standard rapid-sequence induction should then be performed, using intravenous sodium thiopentone (2–4 mg per kg of a 2.5 per cent solution) given over 20–30 seconds, or intravenous etomidate (100–300 mg per kg) followed by intravenous suxamethonium chloride (1.0 1.5 mg per kg). Muscle fasciculation commonly occurs within 30–90 seconds, and is followed by complete voluntary-muscle paralysis. Intubation is then performed as described above.

For patients requiring positive-pressure ventilation and continued muscle-paralysis, a non-depolarizing agent such as pancuronium bromide in a dosage of 4–8 mg should be given. Failure to intubate a patient who has been paralysed with suxamethonium necessitates bag-and-mask ventilation until the effect of the muscle relaxant has worn off. This is usually within 5–10 minutes.

Neither the induction nor the paralysing drugs mentioned above provide analgesia or sedation. This must be given where appropriate, using a suitable opioid (for example, phenoperidine 2–5 mg) and a benzodiazepine (for example, diazepam 10–20 mg or midazolam 2.5–7.5 mg).

Suxamethonium chloride is a depolarizing neuromuscular blocking drug which may cause acute rises in plasma-potassium. Accordingly it should not be used in patients with severe burns or crush injuries.

Following intubation a chest X-ray should be obtained to confirm the position of the E-T tube. Because of the acute angle between the right main-stem bronchus and trachea, right main-stem intubation is common when an endotracheal tube is inserted too far distally. This can usually be prevented by positioning the 22 cm marker of the endotracheal tube such that it coincides with the upper teeth.

Arterial blood-gas analysis should then be performed to ensure that adequate oxygenation and ventilation are being achieved.

Nasotracheal intubation

Potential advantages of this technique are that it can be performed in patients who are spontaneously breathing, or those in whom movement of the cervical spine is contraindicated. However, epistaxis is a common complication. The size of the endotracheal tube used will be smaller than for the oral route, and the success rates are significantly lower.

If possible, topical cocaine or adrenalin applied to the nasal mucosa may reduce the risk of epistaxis.

The head is placed in the neutral position, and the tip of the lubricated endotracheal tube is placed into the nostril and advanced into the oropharynx (Fig. 10.14).

In spontaneously breathing patients, respiratory sounds may be heard as the tip of the E-T tube approaches the glottic opening.

With a single movement, the tube is then advanced into the trachea during inspiration.

Nasotracheal intubation can be performed under direct vision with a laryngoscope. The tip of the endotracheal tube is grasped with McGill forceps and guided under direct vision through the vocal cords into the trachea.

The cuff of the endotracheal tube is then inflated, cricoid pressure is released, and the tube is secured to the face.

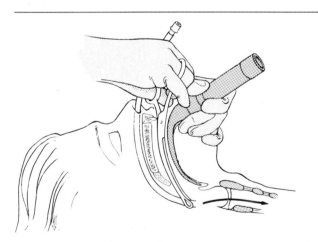

Fig. 10.14 • Advanced airway management 3: nasotracheal intubation

Needle Cricothyrotomy

Surgical approaches to the airway are extremely rarely required in the emergency room. Situations where this may be considered include major injury to the face or oropharynx, or inability to achieve endotracheal intubation via the oral or nasal route. For patients *in extremis*, the use of needle cricothyrotomy is recommended, prior to performing formal cricothyrotomy.

The skin overlying the cricoid and thyroid cartilages is cleaned with antiseptic. The cricothyroid membrane is palpable between the thyroid and the cricoid cartilages.

A large-bore (10–12 FG) needle-cannula assembly is inserted in the mid-line through the skin and the cricothyroid membrane into the trachea (Fig. 10.15).

It is helpful to aspirate as the needle and cannula are advanced. Entry to the trachea is associated with ability to aspirate air. The needle is gently withdrawn, while the cannula is advanced downwards into the trachea.

Intermittent ventilation can be performed using a Y-connector attached to an oxygen supply at 15 litres per minute.

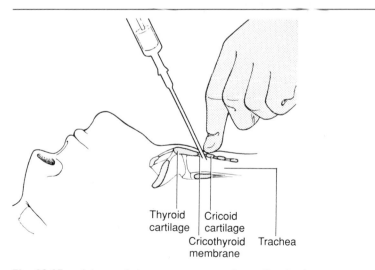

Thyroid | Cricoid
cartilage | cartilage
Cricothyroid   Trachea
membrane

Fig. 10.15 • Advanced airway management 4: needle cricothyrotomy

Ventilation is then applied by placing a thumb over the open end of the Y-connector, in a ratio of 1 second of occlusion to 4 seconds off.

Adequate oxygenation can be maintained for short periods (20–40 minutes) using this technique.

Possible complications include local haematoma-formation and injury to the posterior wall of the trachea or oesophagus if the assembly is introduced too far.

Surgical cricothyroidotomy

Where the patient's condition allows, the area over the cricothyroid membrane is anaesthetized with 1 per cent plain lignocaine. It is helpful to stabilize the thyroid cartilage with the left hand.

With the scalpel held in the right hand make a 2–3 cm-long horizontal incision over the cricothyroid membrane. The membrane is then incised (Fig. 10.16).

It is helpful to insert the handle of the scalpel into the incision and rotate it through 90° to open the airway.

An appropriately-sized cuffed endotracheal or tracheostomy tube may then be introduced through the incision in the cricothyroid membrane, directing the tube distally into the trachea (Fig. 10.17).

The cuff of the endotracheal tube is then inflated. If an obturator is present in the tracheostomy tube, this is removed, and the patient is then ventilated.

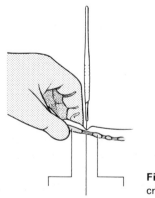

Fig. 10.16 • Advanced airway management 5: cricothyroidotomy 1: incision site

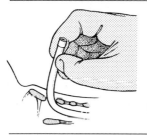

Fig. 10.17 • Advanced airway management 6:
cricothyroidotomy 2: insertion of tube

The tube must be carefully anchored to the patient by tapes
and/or sutures, to prevent dislodgement.

Resuscitation Room thoracotomy

This technique is for experienced personnel only. Appropriate
back-up facilities in relation to surgical personnel and theatre-
access must be available.

Acute pericardial tamponade is the primary indication for this
technique. This will usually be for the patient with a penetrating
wound to the thorax who arrives in the Emergency Department
warm, but with no vital signs.

Occasionally, for individuals skilled in the technique and with
appropriate back-up facilities, cross-clamping of the descending
aorta may be life-saving for patients with exsanguinating intra-
abdominal injuries.

An incision is made from just lateral to the sternum to the mid-
axillary line in the fifth left intercostal space (Fig. 10.18). In female
patients the incision should be in the submammary fold. The
pectoralis major, serratus anterior, and intercostal muscles are
divided, and the pleura is visualized. Since these patients are in
'cardiac arrest', little in the way of bleeding should be encountered.

The pleura is incised, and a self-retaining rib-spreader is
inserted into the incision and opened, allowing direct access to the
pleural cavity.

The lung is retracted in a posterior and lateral direction, and the
pericardium and heart will then be visualized.

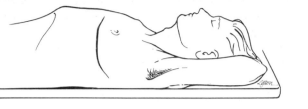

Fig. 10.18 • Thoracotomy 1: incision site

The percardial sac should be incised longitudinally, taking care that the left phrenic nerve is not divided (Fig. 10.19).

Blood or clots in the pericardial sac are removed. Initially bleeding from penetrating wounds to the heart should be controlled by direct digital pressure, and if no spontaneous cardiac activity is present internal cardiac massage should be performed. Penetrating heart-wounds should not normally be sutured in the Resuscitation Room, as this technique is often difficult, and can lead to further myocardial damage. In general, direct digital pressure provides better control from the bleeding-site than clamping or the insertion of a Foley catheter, with the balloon subsequently inflated with saline and gentle traction

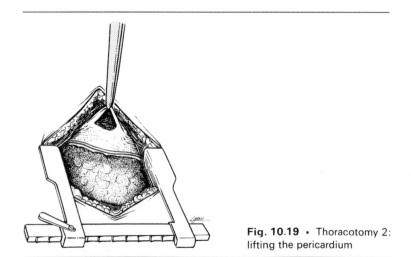

Fig. 10.19 • Thoracotomy 2: lifting the pericardium

applied. Where internal cardiac massage is required, a two-handed technique should be used, taking care to avoid further injury to the thin-walled atria.

Compression of the heart should be performed at the rate of 60–80 per minute, while rapid volume-replacement and resuscitation are continued.

Bleeding from the intercostal vessels or internal mammary arteries are rarely a problem in the initial stages, when cardiac output is absent or drastically reduced. However when the procedure begins to be successful, bleeding from intercostal or internal mammary arteries may be brisk and require prompt clamping and ligation.

Following these emergency measures the patient who has regained cardiac output should be transferred directly to the operating theatre for further formal exploration and definitive care.

Further reading

Champion, H. R., Robb, J. V., and Trunkey, D. D. (ed.) (1989). Robb and Smith's operative surgery, 4th edn. Trauma surgery, part 1. Butterworth, London.

Fosse, E., Svennevig, J.-L., Larsen, J. P., Gerrer, T., and Westrup, J. (1989). Human immunodeficiency virus and hepatitis B virus in injured patients and victims of violence. Injury, 20, 13–15.

Rosen, P. and Sternback, G. (ed.) (1983). Atlas of emergency medicine, 2nd edn. Williams & Wilkins, Baltimore/London.

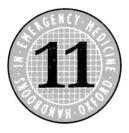

Last things

Last things: the 'human' dimension

• **A medical challenge The human being Reassurance of the patient Trauma Team leaders The patient's relatives Facing up to death Involving the GP Staff counselling**

The management of the multiply injured patient from the scene of accident to subsequent rehabilitation or death is one of the most complex and challenging of medical situations.

In the frenetic activity of the Resuscitation Room, with the patient undergoing a multitude of diagnostic and therapeutic interventions, it can be all too easy to lose sight of the human being at the centre of the activity.

While a proportion of patients sustaining multiple injury will have altered or complete loss of consciousness, many will be fully sentient and aware. They will frequently be in pain, distressed, and fearful of dying. These factors will be aggravated by the unfamiliarity of the environment, the personnel, and the procedures which they are undergoing.

All patients require to be reassured and comforted, and where procedures are being undertaken explanation must be given. Even where a patient is thought to have altered or lost consciousness, the behaviour, manner, and tone of people in the Resuscitation Room should always be such as to provide reassurance to such patients.

Repeatedly in this book we have emphasized the importance of having senior experienced staff involved from the outset in the management of these patients. Only in this way can the patient be managed expeditiously, and with no inter-speciality wrangling as to priority or access to the patient. Discussions regarding further investigation and management must *never* be conducted over a patient lying on a trolley in the Resuscitation Room. The specialist teams involved, under the direction of the Trauma Team leader, must rapidly formulate an individual management-plan for each patient, and arrange for it to be put into practice without delay.

In our experience the Trauma Team leader needs to be of the seniority of a Senior Registrar or Consultant for such liaison and specialist team guidance to be performed optimally. The conduct of the Team leader within the Resuscitation Room can lend much to the efficiency and speed at which the various processes will be performed. His voice should never need to be raised. The most efficient, structured, and rapid resuscitation will occur with little in the way of extraneous noise and under the calm, controlled direction of such an individual.

The patient is at the tip of a pyramid of people affected by his injuries. The patient's relatives and friends will often arrive with the patient or shortly after the patient has arrived in the Emergency Department. Adequate facilities for their reception must be available.

These should include a secluded, quiet room with comfortable chairs, refreshments, and the ability to make outside telephone calls.

The patient's relatives must be kept as fully informed as possible, given the uncertain and often rapidly changing situation. This task is frequently delegated to the most junior members of the medical and nursing staff team—a practice which is to be deplored.

When speaking to relatives, information must be given slowly, and where possible using non-technical language. Judgemental comments and opinions as to the events preceding or related to the accident itself must be avoided.

Relatives often have only one question—'Is he going to live, doctor?' This question can rarely be answered directly, and a combination of honesty and tact are necessary. The prognosis for an individual patient following multiple injury is rarely predictable at this early stage. To falsely raise or dash relatives' hopes can be devastating, and can lead to major problems subsequently. However, an indication of the gravity of the patient's situation should be conveyed, together with the likely sequence of further events over the next few hours, for example surgery or transfer to a specialized unit.

Where transfer is to occur, arrangements for the relatives to follow (rather than accompany) the patient should be made. At the receiving centre, relatives should be met, and further information should be provided by the team that will be undertaking future care. Where a trauma patient dies in the Resuscitation Room or the Emergency Department, the situation can be even more complex. The relatives will often have rushed to hospital having little expectation or knowledge of the severity of the event, and will be unprepared for such news. The normal doctor–patient–relative *rapport* will not have been made, and inept or clumsy handling at this difficult time can make the later grieving process for relatives even more difficult. The most senior doctor and nurse who have been involved in the patient's care should normally perform this task. Euphemisms such as 'passed on' or 'slipped away' should not be used. The relatives must clearly, but compassionately, be told that the patient has died. Otherwise, processes of denial or misunderstanding can occur.

Where appropriate, additional religious requirements, such as 'The Sacrament of the Sick' will be required, and the help of chaplains, priests, rabbis, and others can be invaluable. The relatives may wish to see the body of the deceased patient. Except in rare or extreme circumstances, where such gross disfiguration or mutilation have occurred that it is considered that this would cause additional grief, such requests should not be denied. The sight of the dead loved one, and the ability to touch, kiss, and hold the body, will help the 'normal' progression of the bereavement process.

The patient's general practitioner must always be contacted as soon as possible. This will provide additional support and assistance for the family. Medications, such as 'sleeping tablets' or sedatives, should not be given to relatives, as this will blunt the normal bereavement process, and may lead to iatrogenic problems. Where pharmacological assistance is required, it should be provided on a short-term basis, carefully monitored by the patient's own general practitioner.

The relatives must have a clearly identified individual who they can contact in the event of further questions or concerns arising. It is best for this information to be written or printed on paper for the relatives, with the hospital's telephone number, and the individual's name, designation, and extension.

Finally, the effects of these cases on medical, nursing, and ancillary staff involved in their initial reception and resuscitation are often neglected. The exposure to patients suffering pain or mutilation, and to death, can be devastating for unsupported staff of all grades.

Regular meetings of staff involved in major trauma cases for the purposes of audit are *not* the occasion for such support to be provided. Our own experience is that formal 'counselling' is of less value than the ability of members of the team to support each other in an informal manner. With sensitively given support and encouragement given mutually, the team can be enriched by these experiences, and can identify those areas where improvements can be made in the reception of future patients.

Further reading

Rosen, P. and Honigman, B. (1988). Life and death. In *Emergency medicine—concepts and clinical practice*, 2nd edn, ed. P. Rosen, 5–26. Mosby, St Louis.

Appendix

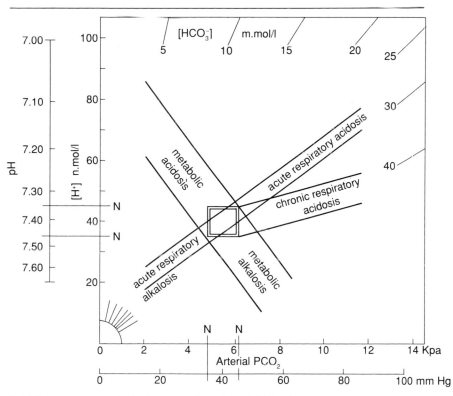

Acid–base nomogram in the interpretation of arterial blood-gases

Index